MUSCLE YOUR WAY
THROUGH MENOPAUSE
...and Beyond

ALSO BY JUDITH SHERMAN-WOLIN

Smart Girls Do Dumbbells

MUSCLE YOUR WAY
THROUGH MENOPAUSE
...and Beyond

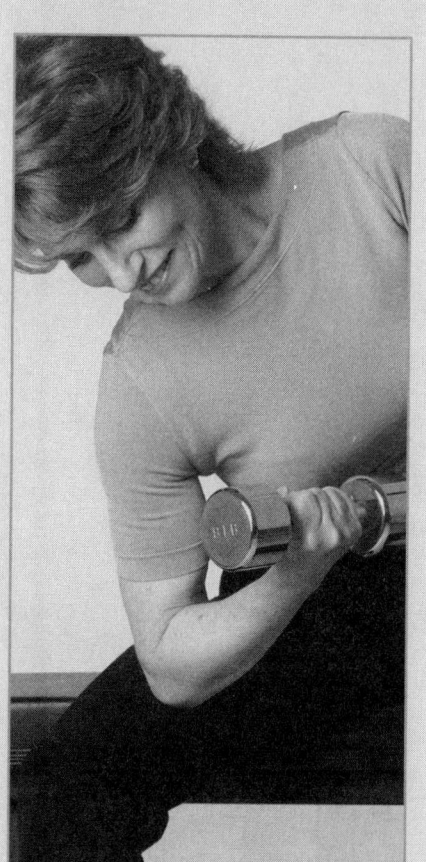

10 Anti-Aging Exercise Strategies for a **Leaner,** **Younger,** **Sexier Future**

JUDITH SHERMAN-WOLIN,
ACSM H/FI, NSCA-CPT

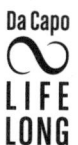

Da Capo
LIFE LONG

A Member of the Perseus Books Group
New York

Printed in the United States of America.
Da Capo Press is a member of the Perseus Books Group

Text design by BackStory Design
Set in 11.75 point Adobe Garamond

ISBN 10: 0-7382-1077-3
ISBN 13: 978-0-7382-1077-3

First printing, January 2007

Da Capo Press books are available at special discounts for bulk purchases in the U.S. by corporations, institutions, and other organizations. For more information, please contact the Special Markets Department at the Perseus Books Group, 11 Cambridge Center, Cambridge, MA 02142, or email special.markets@perseusbooks.com.

For Samantha and Bennett,
who make the journey priceless
and the rewards endless.

CONTENTS

SECTION ONE

THE ANTI-AGING STRATEGIES

SECTION TWO

THE 6-WEEK BODY & HEALTH RECLAMATION PROGRAMS

FOREWORD

Over the past century, the life span of women has changed dramatically. About a third of a woman's life will be spent in menopause. While this natural biological transition can be well managed by most women, it is a time of profound physiological changes.

The cessation of ovarian function, with the loss of estrogen and progesterone, along with physiological aging of the body, results in changes in the skeleton and muscles that support it and the healthy function of most vital organ systems. Degenerative diseases, weakness, metabolic and cardiovascular diseases, all accelerate from the onset of menopause.

One hundred years ago few women lived very much beyond the onset of menopause, and so little was known about the prevention of the changes women were experiencing. Today, modern science has allowed us to understand and treat many of the degenerative changes occurring in aging women. More drugs are being developed for osteoporosis, hypercholesterolemia, heart failure, and depression. In addition, the medical gurus preach prevention as part of every day living, with diet control, weight loss, and vitamin and mineral therapy. Clearly exercise and physical fitness have become a critical part of this prevention practice. What follows is a book, the first of its kind, to articulate the purpose and methods for the use of exercise specifically aimed at menopausal and post-menopausal women for the maintenance of good health and the prevention and reduction of deterioration that accompanies menopause and aging. Judith Sherman-Wolin is eminently experienced and qualified to help women resist muscle wasting, bone loss, and metabolic alterations with exercise and physical fitness. For those of us in the practice of medicine and dealing with large numbers of menopausal women, we now have an adjunctive device, *Muscle Your Way Through Menopause . . . and Beyond,* to help us prevent these degenerative diseases.

Philip G. Brooks, M.D.
Clinical Professor, Department of Ob-Gyn,
David Geffen School of Medicine at UCLA
Attending Physician, Cedars-Sinai Medical Center,
Los Angeles, California

INTRODUCTION

It is a mistake to regard age as a downhill grade toward dissolution. The reverse is true. As one grows older, one climbs with surprising strides.

GEORGE SAND

There is possibly no other human biological function that has been as riddled with mythology and mystery, contradiction and confusion than menopause.

In the 1700s, when the earliest written records of menopause are dated, it was diagnosed as an "illness" and "treated" with leeches and bloodletting as a way to purge the body of the "poisonous blood" that was no longer eliminated during menstruation.

Thank goodness scientific discovery came along with the enlightened evidence that it was hormones, not "evil spirits," that regulated women's bodies, putting an end to these barbaric procedures! Still, this natural, normal biological event continues to be rife with controversy and debate. We are confused, sometimes scared, and quite often overwhelmed by conflicting information as how best to face our changing bodies and altering lives.

Even today, with all our scientific knowledge, there remains a belief among some women that menopause is the beginning of the end, signaling the termination of their vitality, vivacity, and sexuality.

I wrote the Anti-Aging Exercise Strategies, listed below, and created the Body Reclamation Programs found in Section Two of this book, to dispel these myths. These Anti-Aging Strategies teach you the muscle physiology of your body and exercise techniques that will help you preserve and maintain a healthy, beautiful, functional body throughout the aging process.

Anti-Aging Exercise Strategy 1
　Structuring Your Strength:
　Muscle's Body- and Health-Preserving Power

Anti-Aging Exercise Strategy 2
　Heart of the Matter
　Cardiovascular

Anti-Aging Exercise Strategy 3
　"Legs" to Stand On
　Movers and Shapers

Anti-Aging Exercise Strategy 4
　Behind the Scenes: "Hip" and "Buttocks"
　Smoothers and Lifters

Anti-Aging Exercise Strategy 5
　Treasure Your "Chest"
　Builders and Boosters

Anti-Aging Exercise Strategy 6
　"Back" in Business
　Reinforcers and Developers

Anti-Aging Exercise Strategy 7
　Up in "Arms"
　Definers and Refiners

Anti-Aging Exercise Strategy 8
　Straight from the "Shoulder"
　Enhancers and Strengtheners

Anti-Aging Exercise Strategy 9
　Hard Core: Flatter "Abs" and Stronger "Back" Forever More

Anti-Aging Exercise Strategy 10
   Stretching Your Body and Balancing Your Life

The Life Balancing Exercises®

The Anti-Aging Workout Systems in Section Two: Your Body and Health Reclamation Programs are designed so that you can select the appropriate program to meet your health and physical needs, and achieve the results you desire.

- Goal: Weight Loss, Tone, and Firm
- Goal: Increase Strength, Tone, and Firm
- Goal: Cardiovascular Health, Tone, and Firm

If you are seriously committed to the programs and sincerely believe you deserve the gift of good health and a quality lifestyle, and follow the Anti-Aging Strategies in this book, you will quickly realize chronological aging does not inevitably coincide with the physical deterioration of your body! Sure, just like in the old black and white movies, the calendar pages flip by, birthday candles accumulate and body chemistry changes, but deteriorating health and an aging body are not the inevitable outcome of the passage of time. And I am not alone in my belief. Science and clinical studies back me up.

Dr. Margaret Burghardt, a researcher at the Fowler-Kennedy Sports Medicine Clinic in London, Ontario, Canada, reports, "Even at menopause, fitness can reduce the risk of heart disease, osteoporosis, and diabetes, yet only 38% of women over the age of 19 exercise regularly."

And what about the inevitable weight gain and loss of physical strength we often associate with the onset of menopause? One seminal study on the effects of exercise training on lean and fat mass in women, reported in the *Journal of Gerontology*, states, "Menopause is associated with decreases in lean mass and increases in fat mass. We found significant effects of exercise on increases in total body, arm and leg lean soft tissue mass and decreases in leg fat mass and percentage of body fat."

Over the course of my professional career as a clinical exercise specialist associated with the UCLA Center for Human Nutrition, a fitness editor and consultant, private trainer and lecturer, author and health-fitness activist, I have encountered hundreds of women who have spent a good deal of their lives and time questioning the physical health and beauty of their bodies. I have worked with women of all ages, overweight women and breast cancer survivors, those suffering from diabetes, osteoporosis and metabolic disease, and in my experience with all these women from every walk of life and under every conceivable circumstance, not a single one has ever denied that exercise has improved their lives, health, self-esteem, mood, and of course, their bodies in the most profound and rewarding way.

Maybe some of the reasons you have been reluctant to start protecting your health and body through an age-appropriate exercise program are because you:

- Are intimidated.
- Don't really understand muscle's health value and beauty benefits.
- Don't know where to begin.
- Don't know the proper way to do it.
- Can't get motivated.
- Can't stay with a program.
- Think building muscle means gaining bulk.
- Think it's too late in life.

The Anti-Aging Exercise Strategies and the customized "6-Week Body & Health Reclamation Programs" I write about in this book will help change all that. If you follow the strategies and the program targeted to achieve your personal fitness goals, you will:

- Lose weight.
- Decrease your risk for heart disease, colon cancer, and possibly other life-threatening cancers and diseases.

- Gain muscle.
- Preserve bone.
- Increase your range of motion and flexibility.
- Gain energy.
- Improve your mood.
- Increase your self-esteem.
- Feel more vibrant and alive.
- Improve the quality of your life throughout the aging process.

As you start applying the Anti-Aging Exercise Strategies, you begin a life-altering journey. Your destination is improved health, increased physical strength, and a leaner, more beautiful body. Along with the physical and physiological improvements come wonderful surprises you probably never associated with exercise and physical fitness: emotional balance, confidence and pride, serenity, and a renewed sense of well-being.

Please join me now for this transforming odyssey into a future of healthy aging, longevity, and beauty as you *Muscle Your Way Through Menopause . . . and Beyond.*

SECTION ONE

THE ANTI-AGING STRATEGIES

Structuring Your Strength

Muscle's Body- And Health-Preserving Power

Generally speaking, women underrate their physical strength.

MILTON

Muscle is miracle tissue and can impact your body and your spirit in a life-preserving way, especially as you traverse the menopausal passage. It is anti-aging, health-promoting, and life-enhancing. It helps you stay stronger, healthier, more youthful, vibrant and vigorous, while combating the physical and emotional signs and symptoms of menopause. It can help revitalize your confidence, power, and pride.

However, not many women appreciate or really understand the importance of a body composition rich in muscle. A perfect example is Jane. E. Brody, the highly regarded health writer from the *New York Times*. In an article she wrote in 1999 entitled, "For Younger Muscles, Just Pump Away," she says, "I was a bit taken aback when an exercise physiologist asked if I did any form of strength training. Don't my regular activities keep me as strong as I'm likely to get?"

The answer, she discovered, was no. Even though Ms. Brody, at the age of 58 when the article was written, was highly physically active through walking, tennis, swimming, biking, and ice skating, she discovered her arms weren't even strong enough to do biceps curls with a two-pound dumbbell. This was her awakening: "Many people have shunned the idea of muscle-building exercises because they harbor misconceptions about what it is, whom it is for and what it does to the body."

These "misconceptions" are primarily true of women. "For the vast majority of women, strength training offers an opportunity to reduce flab and improve appearance without detracting one iota from femininity," wrote Ms. Brody.

But it's not just about reducing flab. There are profound health and life-altering benefits to strength training and building muscle through exercise that are especially critical to ensure a healthy aging process for the menopausal woman.

Margaret Burghardt, a staff physician at the Fowler-Kennedy Sports Medicine Clinic, University of Western Ontario Faculty of Medicine, believes even at menopause, fitness can reduce your risk of heart disease, osteoporosis, and diabetes.

In an article entitled, "Exercise at Menopause: A Critical Difference," she writes, "From age 35 onwards, women lose bone mass at a rate of about 0.75% to 1% per year and the loss increases to 2% to 3% per year at menopause, most markedly from the lumbar spine."

She cites one study in which menopausal women showed an increase in lumbar spine bone mineral density (BMD) of 3.5% in women who exercised whereas BMD in the controls decreased 2.7%, suggesting that exercise can inhibit or reverse the osteoporosis associated with aging.

She goes on to report, "Even in the elderly woman, exercise can attenuate certain effects of aging and sedentary lifestyles. Regular exercise may decrease the incidence and severity of hot flashes, which occur in 75% of menopausal women.

"Weight-bearing exercise, resistance training and high-intensity fitness regimens can reduce a woman's risk of fractures," she also documents.

Dr. Burghardt is just one of a growing number of physicians and clinical researchers who are discovering and prescribing weight bearing exercise and weight resistance training to women dealing with the impact of menopause on their health and their bodies. While our bodies do change throughout the aging process, Dr. Burghardt is saying that these physical and physiological changes can be mitigated by the choices we make and the course of action we pursue everyday on behalf of ourselves.

MUSCLE LOSS THROUGHOUT THE AGES

Muscle accounts for 45% of your body weight, but its mass declines with advancing age. From the ages of 20 to 90, adults lose about 50% of their muscle mass, and with this loss their strength declines by about 15% each decade after 50.

The typical woman starts losing about one percent of muscle mass each year by her late thirties and early forties and gains that amount in body fat. In the absence of progressive resistance training, muscle loss increases with each decade:

- 5% per decade from the age of 50.
- 10% from the age of 70.
- 20% from the age of 80.

Loss of muscle mass presents serious health and lifestyle concerns, especially for women. Data from a Framingham study indicates 45% of women ages 65 to 74 and 65% of women ages 75 to 84 cannot lift a 10-pound dumbbell.

Along with this decline in strength and muscle, your body changes both physically and physiologically.

Below are many of the important health benefits you can expect to realize when you follow the Anti-Aging Exercise Strategies and Anti-Aging Workout Systems presented in *Muscle Your Way Through Menopause . . . and Beyond*:

Muscle loss

⇩

Slowdown of your metabolism

⇩

Decline in your functional mobility

(Walking, getting up out of a chair, freedom of movement)

⇩

Decline in your confidence

⇧

Inactivity

⇧

Increase in your risk for heart disease, some cancers, including breast and colon

⇧

Obesity

⇧

Risk for type 2 diabetes, lower back pain, chronic diseases

- Reduce your risk for heart disease (which currently kills more women than men in this country).
- Reduce your risk for some types of cancer, including breast and colon cancer.
- Reduce your risk for developing type 2 diabetes. Muscle is the largest repository for glucose in the body. Blood-glucose levels tend to rise as muscle diminishes throughout the aging process and inactivity escalates.
- Increase your HDL (good cholesterol) and slow the rate of increase in LDL cholesterol.
- Prevent weight gain, especially increases in intra-abdominal fat.
- Improvement in blood pressure.

- Reduce your risk for increasingly losing bone mass (osteopinia and osteoporosis) throughout the aging process because muscle exerts force on bones and helps build bone density (similar to the effects of HRT, but with none of the unwanted side effects). From the Netherlands, a meta-analysis, concludes that post-menopausal women who exercise regularly (including strength training) reduce or reverse bone loss by one percent per year.
- Reduce some of your menopausal symptoms, like hot flashes and fatigue.
- Reduce your risk of arthritis as muscle helps cushion joints.
- Reduction in bouts of depression. One study conducted at Tufts University by investigator Nalin Singh on older adults with moderate depression found dramatic decreases in depression and significant mood improvement in a group that participated in strength training versus a control group that simply received health education.

If the above weren't inspiring enough to get you motivated (and keep you motivated), there are amazing beauty benefits you can expect to realize by following a consistent and intelligent program of exercise, including muscle strengthening:

- A more youthful appearance.
- A leaner looking, sexier body.
- Increased metabolism to help prevent weight gain.
- Strong joints and ligaments.
- Greater energy.
- A more lively and vibrant demeanor.
- Some studies show exercise may also help improve skin elasticity and tone.

This is a formidable list. Yet, with all there is to gain and nothing to lose (except some body fat), many women still possess a fear of following a program of strength training. Following are the fears and concerns I hear most often in my practice:

BUILDING MUSCLE: FEARS AND REALITIES

"I Don't Want Big Muscles."

Lynda's fear: "If I lift weights, I will develop big, bulky muscles. I don't want to look like a man."

Judith: "It is impossible for you to build muscle the same as a man. You will build lean, beautiful muscles that will give you a youthful, healthful-looking body."

Lynda is a pretty, forty-five year-old mother of three. Her concern about building "manly" muscles is not unusual. Many women harbor the same misconception but you cannot develop the same muscular structure as a man (unless you are using performance and muscle enhancing steroids), and here is why: your body doesn't manufacture enough of the required hormone, testosterone, to create the kind of muscle hypertrophy (growth) that men develop. Some researchers estimate that men have twenty to thirty times higher testosterone levels than women, which exerts a significant an-abolic (or tissue building) effect. Women do have the capability to develop strength improvements similar to men, but without the added levels of testosterone, the same type of muscle growth is simply not possible.

"I'm Too Old."

Liz's fear: "I am sixty-seven years old . . . I'm too old to start building muscle."

Judith: "Let me check my exercise physiology book to confirm that fact. . . nope, no mention of ever being too old to build muscle—or do anything else you desire to do, for that matter."

Muscle does not age- or gender- discriminate. For example, one semi-nal study, conducted at Tufts University in Boston, involving ten nursing home residents with an average age of ninety, observed a 174% increase in knee extension strength, from twenty to forty-four pounds.

I work with a woman in her early eighties whose strength gains are remarkable. When we started working together, she could only lift three-pound dumbbells to do her biceps curls. Within three months, she was using fives, and not long thereafter, sevens. These results are not unusual. Additionally, once she started on a regular and consistent exercise program with me, her back and shoulder pain all but disappeared.

As she became physically stronger, she also gained confidence in her body movements. She was no longer fearful of falling because her leg strength increased as her muscles developed strength. She also accomplished one of her major goals: to be able to get up out of a chair without struggling.

"I'm Too Weak."

Susan's fear: "I can't possibly pick that up," she says, pointing to the ten-pound dumbbell on the weight rack.

Judith: "I'm not asking you to pick up that one, I am asking you to pick up this one, its little brother," as I hand her a three-pounder. "And I promise you this; it won't be long before you'll be moving up the weight rack towards that ten-pounder."

Susan looked at me like I had seven eyes, and not all in a row! Like most women, she didn't realize just how much physical strength she possessed. When we started working together to help her build up muscle at the age of fifty-one, she confessed she'd only touched dumbbells to move them out of the way of the vacuum when cleaning her teenage son's bedroom. A single, working mother, she didn't have a lot of extra time, so I created a home-based exercise prescription for her. Within six months, Susan had lost seventeen pounds of body fat, had increased her strength to the point where she was able to do biceps curls with eight-pound dumbbells, and was walking two to three miles five times a week.

Her lower back pain had all but disappeared and she had a new boyfriend. (I am not taking credit for the boyfriend, just the weight loss and strength gains!)

"I Won't Lose Weight If I Build Muscle."

Beth's concern: I have heard a pound of muscle weighs more than a pound of fat so if I build muscle, I won't lose weight."

Judith: "A pound of muscle weighs a pound. A pound of fat also weighs, well, a pound," I tell Beth.

But this is one of those misconceptions I hear all the time and here is the confusion: muscle does weigh more than fat, but since it is much denser it makes the body appear smaller, or thinner, if you will. The reason muscle weighs more is because the muscle cells contain mostly contracticle proteins, primarily myosin and actin, in a watery solution. Fat cells are composed primarily of oils (lipids), which are less dense than water. This is demonstrated every time you mix oil and water. For instance, if you're preparing a salad dressing and you let it stand, what eventually floats to the top? The oil—because it is lighter than the water. So, after training for nine weeks, when Beth asked, "I've only lost a couple of pounds but my clothes are so much looser. Is this possible?" The answer is "yes" because on your body, a pound of fat looks like a ball of yarn whereas a pound of muscle looks like a strand of twine.

"I Have To Belong To a Gym To Exercise Properly."

Lillian's complaint: "I don't like gyms. They are intimidating. And I don't have the time to get there. And they are expensive."

Judith: "True. True. True," I say to Lillian, a sixty-six-year-old woman who takes care of her three grandchildren during the day while their mother is at work. Lillian is active, taking care of her grandchildren, but she is often out of breath, finds it increasingly difficult to lift up the smallest one, and has chronic back problems. Her menopausal symptoms have mostly vanished, but she says she feels she is losing strength with each passing day.

Like Lillian, many women, especially those of us past forty, don't want to go to a gym where it seems as if all the women weigh one-hundred pounds and are a size zero. (The truth is, if you really look around, gyms and commercial fitness facilities are populated with all types, sizes, and shapes of bodies.) But still, there is a fear out there that gyms are the domain of the already fit and fabulous.

This is why over half of the Anti-Aging Exercise Strategies I describe can be done perfectly well at home, with simple and inexpensive equipment. I've even created exercises that require no equipment whatsoever! So, if you think a gym membership is required to lose weight, gain muscle, and become healthier. . . think again!

"I Don't Know Whether I Should Be Using Machines Or Free Weights."

Jane's confusion: "I am not sure if machines are better for me to use than free weights?"

Judith: "Machines are not 'better' than free weights, just a different mechanism for applying resistance to the muscles."

Free weights include dumbbells and barbells and are called "free weights" because they can be fixed to anything, do not require any cables or pulleys, and are easily moved from one location to another. A dumbbell is any weight meant to be lifted in one hand. A barbell is a bar with fixed or changeable weights mounted on each long enough to be gripped with two hands at once.

As a point of information, the origin of the word dumbbell comes from 16th Century Tudor England, where church bells evolved into being lifted by young men to increase muscle size and to demonstrate feats of strength. Apparently, at some point, the noise was too much with all that lifting and clanging, so some innovative young man removed the "clapper" and they became known colloquially as "dumbbells."

More importantly: it is not the equipment you are using. . . but the way in which you are using it. If you use machines incorrectly you run the risk of slow or unwanted results, or even worse, injury, just as if you were using free weights incorrectly.

There are advantages and disadvantages to both.

ADVANTAGES TO MACHINES:

Ease of Use

Some women are more comfortable on machines because they are easier to use. Machines automatically position your body to work the muscle group correctly. Even though you are always responsible to make sure your core is strong and your posture aligned, machines are designed specifically to make certain you are placed in a proper working position.

Safety

Machines can be safer because you don't run the risk of hurting yourself by lifting a dumbbell or barbell improperly. Also, when you are carrying free weights around, you run the risk of dropping them on your foot (or some-one else's.) With machines, you don't have to worry about picking them up, carrying them to your bench or workout area, and re-racking them when you are finished.

Convenience

If you can simply jump on a machine, your workout goes a lot faster. Also, most gyms arrange machines so that if you are doing legs, the leg machines are in a cluster. All the machines that work your back, chest, arms and shoulders are placed near one another so there is less moving around. If you have limited time to spend in the gym, machines offer you the ability to move quickly through your workout.

One last advantage to machines: they also allow you to lift heavier weights. This may be a positive or negative. One of my overriding creeds is: *never sacrifice form for mass*. By this, I mean never lift so heavy that you lose form, risk injury, and delay results. I see lots of people working out in the gym (pardon me, but mainly men!) who are lifting dumbbells that are way too heavy for them to maintain the integrity of the movement. They are asking for injury, especially lower back and neck, and are probably frustrated because they are not attaining their fitness goals due to sloppy form.

ADVANTAGES TO FREE WEIGHTS:

Liberating

As the name implies, they are free, easy to move around. Machines are, well, machines. They are stationary, big, bulky, and it takes a variety of different ones to get through a complete workout. For the most part, they are designed to work one muscle group at a time. You need one for the front of your legs, one for the back of your legs, one to work your chest, biceps, triceps, and shoulders.

When you use free weights, dumbbells, for example, you can get a complete workout with simple equipment you can use at your home, office, or even while on the road. So, you are not confined to a gym to do your workouts.

Results

When you learn to use free weights properly, which I will teach you in the following Anti-Aging Exercise Strategies, you have a greater chance of achieving the results you want faster because you become responsible for your own body integrity. Machines set you up in the way they are designed, not necessarily for how *you* are designed. They can't possibly fit accurately all body lengths, widths, and range of motion limitations. Traditionally, they move in one plane of motion: front, back, side. Our bodies and limbs are transplanar. We move in several planes at once: front, side, horizontally. Using free weights allows you to move in a more natural way, as you would in your real-life movements.

Machines, because of their restrictive design, confine your movements. Also, free weights are free-wheeling. Machines may not be designed to fit your body, so you may have to strain to complete the moves according to the machine's movements, not your own natural biomechanics.

Inexpensive

Obviously, major pieces of gym equipment are quite costly and mostly found in commercial gyms or big fitness centers. However, if you want to do your workouts at home, or even fill in on the days you aren't able to make it to the gym, you can use a few dumbbells and you will get an equally good workout! Dumbbells cost about a dollar a pound, so you can equip a home gym fairly inexpensively. You don't need a lot of big, complicated, and expensive equipment. Staying healthy and fit can be done in very simple, effective, and rewarding ways. And free weights make this possible for everyone.

Time Saving

Many women simply don't have the time to get to a gym, or as I said before, don't like the atmosphere. By keeping a few pieces of equipment in your home (dumbbells, exercise balls, some elastic bands and tubes) you can create your own home gym without the inconvenience, discomfort, and time involved driving to a gym. We all have many obligations tugging at our time everyday: children, work, family obligations, community service, and we don't have a great deal of that precious commodity: *spare time*. Free weights allow you to work out at home when you want to, without worrying about adding extra commute time to the process.

Whether you choose to use machines or free weights, the critical factor in achieving the results you desire is your personal commitment to doing the exercises correctly and consistently.

. . . AND THEN, THERE'S JUDITH'S SIGNATURE NO-EQUIPMENT-NEEDED EXERCISES!

I hear lots of reasons why people can't get started working out or why they can't get to their workouts. There're lots of popular excuses like, "the cat ate my dumbbells" or "my boyfriend ran away with my exercise ball."

In an effort to plug every possible why-I-can't-exercise hole, I designed a series of exercises that require absolutely no equipment, just you and your body showing up and ready to work.

These are effective, easy, convenient, just-getting-started exercises, exercises you can travel with, exercises you can do at the office, while watching television, some even while flying on a plane (as long as you're not the one flying the plane.)

Some of the most effective and difficult exercises advanced exercisers do are body resistance exercises: push-ups, chin-ups, pull-ups, sit-ups. The challenges doing Equipment Free Exercises are:

- Maintaining good form and posture.
- Concentrating on the isometric contractions.
- Controlling the movements.
- Being mentally connected with your body.

Some of the benefits of the Equipment Free Exercises are:

- You can get started immediately!
- They're always available (it's your body).
- You achieve results.
- They add versatility to your workout routine.

- They offer convenience and flexibility.
- They are the best way to learn proper form and technique.

There are all sorts of ways to *Muscle Your Way Through Menopause . . . and Beyond* and these Equipment Free Exercises are just the jump-start you will need!

— ◇ —

In the following Anti-Aging Exercise Strategies, I write about the techniques to help you build lean, healthful muscles properly; about heart and metabolic health; bone preservation; core strengthening; and how to maintain your flexibility and range of motion. Then, I provide you with three *6-Week, Day-by-Day, Anti-Aging Workout Systems*: one focusing on Weight Loss, one to Increase Strength, Firm, and Tone, and one for Cardiovascular Health.

Our goal is threefold:

- To help you stay healthy, physically fit, youthful, and beautiful beginning and during the menopausal passage and beyond.
- To help you create a body rich in muscle tissue that will impact the quality of your health and life for the rest of your life.
- To guide you with the program designed specifically to achieve your exercise and fitness goals for now, and forever.

"*Structuring Your Strength*" is both a physical and spiritual quest; a journey into living a future based on health, strength, and power.

DEGREE OF DIFFICULTY TABLE

In order to help you evaluate what exercises will work for you, I've designed the Degree of Difficulty Grid. It is a simple way to select the appropriate exercises for your needs and fitness level. If you are at a Level One Dumbbell—Slightly Challenging—after a while, when you feel ready, try going to the next level—Two Dumbbells, and test your skill and tolerance for those exercises. If you are at a level Three Dumbbell—Highly Challenging, that does not mean you should not be doing Level One Dumbbell exercises. On the contrary, eventually you will want to be incorporating all the exercises from every level into your Anti-Aging Workout System.

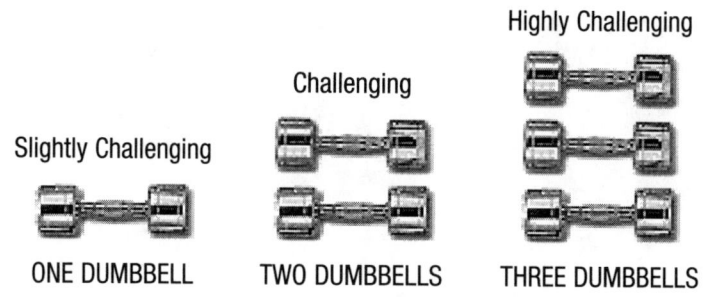

Slightly Challenging
ONE DUMBBELL

Challenging
TWO DUMBBELLS

Highly Challenging
THREE DUMBBELLS

Heart of the Matter
Cardiovascular Health

La distance n'y fait; il n'y a que le premier pas qui coute.
The distance is nothing; it is only the first step that is difficult.

MME. DU DEFFAND

When I taught exercise intervention principles at UCLA, a physician referred a patient to me who was predisposed to coronary artery disease (CAD). She was 51, overweight, suffering from both hypertension and high cholesterol, inactive, and with a family history of CAD.

She came into my gym and before I even had a chance to say "dumbbells" she said, "I hate to exercise. You'll never find a way to make me do it." It was clear, my job wasn't going to be easy. . . but I *love* a challenge and also a convert. We sat down and for the first fifteen minutes we talked about everything *but* exercise. Finally I asked her, "So, tell me, what you do like to do?"

"I like to shop." Good answer, I thought.

We talked a little longer—she, still unconvinced a consultation with me would in any way alter her inherent dislike of exercise; I, determined to find a way. I listened to her arguments and her complaints about how the doctor said she had to lose weight and her cholesterol and blood pressure were too high, and she was headed for atherosclerosis (a disease involving cholesterol and fatty deposits on the heart's arteries). Not only that, but she couldn't fit into any of her favorite pants anymore and she hated to exercise.

[19]

At long last I offered her the following suggestion, "How about this, I would like you to walk twenty minutes a day, that's it, no more. . . and where I would like you to walk is down Rodeo Drive. You can window shop. It is the perfect place for you to walk." (Rodeo Drive is a fancy street in Beverly Hills where a lot of celebrities shop and the stores are beautiful with interesting and luxurious window displays.)

"You'll be sort of shopping, but without actually stopping to buy anything."

"My husband would love you."

She reluctantly agreed and made an appointment to come see me in a month. When she returned I weighed her in. She had lost about seven pounds. "Wow, that's fantastic. Tell me what you've been doing."

"I started walking, like you said, down Rodeo Drive."

"For twenty minutes each day?"

"Actually, it takes around forty-five minutes, you know, because the new spring collections came in and there's a lot to see."

I spent the next hour showing her some simple weight training exercises she could do at home to build and tone her weakened muscles, how to do abdominal work to help flatten her tummy area, and a few important stretches. The entire routine wouldn't take more than twenty-five minutes.

When she came back to see me, six months later, she had lost close to twenty pounds, had gained muscle, had an improved bone density scan, and her waist had shrunk about two inches. Not only did she look amazing, but her blood pressure and cholesterol were almost normal. Her physician was extremely pleased with her improved health profile. (As was I!)

"Have your feelings about exercise changed over these last six months?" I asked.

"Nope. Every day it's a struggle. But I'll never give it up now. I can fit into my skinny pants. I'm healthier. I look like I did 10 years ago and I feel amazing. You tricked me," she smiled.

I smiled as well.

EXERCISE DURING AND AFTER THE MENOPAUSAL YEARS: ITS IMPORTANCE AND IMPACT

In Dr. Margaret Burghardt's study I mentioned earlier, she states, "The years surrounding the menopause, which occurs at an average age of 52, when a woman undergoes the transition from a reproductive to a postre-productive state, are termed the climacteric period. Regular exercise can prevent, or lessen the impact of many of the changes women experience at this time."

WHAT CONSTITUTES REGULAR EXERCISE AND WHAT EXACTLY SHOULD I BE DOING?

Physicians often tell their patients "you need to go out and exercise," which is an ambiguous prescription at best because the patients have no idea what they're supposed to be doing and most physicians have no idea what to tell them to do. I remember as a child my mother used to say to me, "Go outside and play." And I'd reply, "Play what?" I needed direction.

This is one of the reasons I wanted to write *Muscle Your Way Through Menopause . . . and Beyond.* To give you clear and precise directions on the exercises you need to do, the correct way to do them, and the Anti-Aging Exercise Programs to follow so you know what to do each day.

In this Strategy, I am introducing you to the methods to help you protect your heart through cardiovascular exercise. In the following Strategies, I write about the major muscle groups and give you detailed instructions on how to build and maintain your vital muscle tissue, core strength, and flexibility.

There are two classifications of exercise, anaerobic and aerobic. They are different in this way: "cardiovascular" exercise is "aerobic" exercise while "resistance training" or "muscle retention exercise" is "anaerobic." Both are equally and vitally important to your physical fitness and overall health.

AEROBIC AND ANAEROBIC: WHAT'S THE DIFFERENCE?

So, what exactly is the difference between aerobic and anaerobic exercise, you ask?

Literally, aerobic means "living in air." Simply put, aerobic exercise is an exercise activity during which oxygen is metabolized to produce energy because your body has used up most of its immediately accessible stored energy (glycogen, which is the storage form of glucose in the liver and muscles). It is usually exercise that goes beyond two minutes duration, increases your heart rate and volume of consumed oxygen (Vo_2), and allows you to keep your heart working in a steady state for a duration of time. Examples of aerobic exercises are:

- Walking
- Hiking
- Running
- Aerobic classes
- Kick boxing classes
- Jogging
- Machine-based stair climbing
- Swimming
- Cycling
- Rowing
- Combined arm and leg ergometry
- Dancing
- Skating
- Cross-country skiing
- Jumping rope

Anaerobic means "without oxygen." Anaerobic exercise utilizes stored energy. It is defined as "the short-term energy system." It is exercise that can be completed in short bursts of energy release, between 60 to 180 seconds.

- Resistance Training (lifting weights)
- Tennis
- Golf
- Yoga
- Pilates
- Sprints: 200-meter dash or a 100-meter swim

YOUR CARDIOVASCULAR HEALTH

In practical terms, in the American College of Sports Medicine (ACSM) *Guidelines for Exercise Testing and Prescription*, it suggests the greatest improvements in aerobic fitness occur when exercise involves the *"utilization of large muscle groups in a rhythmic activity over prolonged period of time and aerobic in nature."*

I will break this down for you.

1. Large muscle groups: Your legs. The muscles in the front of your legs, the quadriceps, are the largest muscle group in your body. The muscles in the back of your legs are the hamstrings, also a large muscle group. Another large group of muscles is your gluteals, or buttocks muscles.
2. Rhythmic: constantly recurring sequence of repetitive movements walking, running, jogging, stair-climbing, swimming, and biking.
3. Prolonged period of time: From 10 to 60 minutes.
4. Aerobic in nature—an activity that increases your heart rate and keeps it in a steady state between 60% to 90% of your maximum heart rate.

Your maximal heart rate (MHR) is based upon your age. The formula to calculate your MHR is very simple:

220 Minus Your Age

So, if you are fifty years old, your MHR would be 220–50=170 beats per minute. However, in health-fitness activities we only use percentages of our MHR. An example would be, if you want to use 70% of your MHR, you would multiply .70 x 170, which would be 119 beats per minute.

A few of the benefits of a well-designed, consistent cardiovascular program are:

- Heart Health—Helps protect you from developing metabolic diseases—hypertension, high cholesterol, and type 2 diabetes that can lead to cardiovascular disease.
- Weight Loss—Helps you lose weight and create a healthier body composition.
- Hot Flashes—Possibly helps decrease the severity and frequency of hot flashes.
- Bone Protection—Protection of bones and possible prevention of osteoporosis and estoporotic fractures.
- Mood Improvement—Reduction in depression and mood swings.

HEART HEALTH

Your heart. It's the most poetic part of your physical body, hailed and regaled in poetry, love songs, Shakespearean tragedies, and Hollywood follies. But the heart of myth and mythology has little to do with your actual heart muscle, which is relentless in its determination to keep on pumping. In addition to transporting oxygenated blood from your lungs to tissues and deoxygenated blood from the tissues back to your lungs, your heart and its over 60,000 miles of blood vessels (your cardiovascular system) distributes nutrients, removes metabolic wastes, transports hormones and enzymes, maintains fluid volume preventing dehydration, and helps maintain body temperature by absorbing and redistributing heat. It is about the size of your fist and weighs between 250 and 350 grams. To give you some idea, 455 grams is about one pound. So this mighty muscle is heroic in its serious-minded business of keeping you alive.

According to the National Heart, Lung and Blood Institute (NHLBI), part of the National Institute of Health, U.S. Department of Health and Human Services, "Heart disease is the number one killer of American women, but many women do not realize they are at risk."

Furthermore, the NHLBI notes the time when a woman's risk of heart disease begins to rise is between the ages of 40 to 60. Studies reveal the loss of estrogen during menopause does seem to be a factor in increasing your risk for heart disease, although they are not sure why. But decreases in estrogen alone are not the culprit. Other risk factors include:

- Smoking
- Overweight and obesity
- High blood pressure
- High blood cholesterol
- Physical inactivity
- Diabetes
- Genetics
- Age

The NHBLI emphasizes in its literature that only family history and age are beyond your control. You can prevent or control most of the other factors that increase your risk for heart disease. And one of those preventative measures is pursuing a course of aerobic activity on a daily basis.

As far as selecting a mode of aerobic exercise, you have lots of choices, as listed above, to fulfill the cardiovascular component of your exercise program. Is any one better than the other? Absolutely not. It's a completely personal choice based on your fitness level, limitations due to any injuries, and personal likes or dislikes.

My favorite is walking (although I love tango dancing as well). I like walking for the following reasons:

- Always available (it goes where you go!).
- Inexpensive (two feet, no membership fee).
- Doesn't take a lot of fancy or expensive equipment (except good walking shoes).
- Convenient (ready to go when you are).
- Results (burns an average of 125 calories per 30 minutes).
- You can walk indoors or out, anytime, anywhere (that's safe).

My daughter, Samantha, likes kickboxing. It's fun and high energy. She's got an intense job and work schedule and if she can't get to her kickboxing class, she has some tapes to fill in at home at night or early morning.

I have some clients who suffer from osteoarthritis so they are most comfortable doing their workouts in the swimming pool because it doesn't place any stress on their joints. Swimming is an excellent exercise, but a word of caution: it is a non-weight bearing exercise. As is biking. So, if you are osteopenic (pre-estoporotic) or if you already suffer from osteoporosis, a gravity-based exercise, walking or hiking, is a better choice for you to help with bone mineralization (bone growth and preservation).

WEIGHT BEARING VERSUS WEIGHT RESISTANCE EXERCISES

This is another question I'm frequently asked: what is the difference between weight bearing exercise and weight resistance exercise? Weight bearing exercise is an exercise in which your own body weight is used against gravity—like walking, jogging, and running. Weight resistance exercises are the ones that use some sort of mechanism of applied resistance (dumbbells, exercise bands, machines) against your muscles to help them grow and get stronger. The Anti-Aging Exercises Strategies found in the upcoming chapters are weight resistance exercises to help you build muscle, increase your metabolism so you burn more calories every day, and strengthen your joints and ligaments.

WEIGHT LOSS

It creeps up on you, like a snake in the grass. Menopausal weight gain. Your diet's been pretty much the same and yet suddenly, you're confronted with . . . *mid-body fat.* It's like you've been sideswiped. You didn't even see it coming!

In a study conducted by Wing and colleagues and reported in the Archives of Internal Medicine, the researchers discovered, ". . . body weight in women tends to increase around the time of menopause." This weight gain can actually begin at premenopause, between the ages of 42 to 50 years. The weight gain averages between 5 and 10 pounds. They went on to state, "The women who experienced the greatest weight gain had the lowest exercise levels. . . ."

And here's what their study concluded about exercise: "Exercise has been shown to result in total body weight loss through energy expenditure, a change in the muscle-to-fat ratio, and increased metabolic rate . . . Preservation of muscle mass through endurance and/or resistance training exercise can help to prevent the observed age-related decreases in metabolic rate and overall increase in body fat."

Remember, the more muscle you have, the more calories you burn at rest. It is estimated that a pound of muscle burns approximately 14 calories per twenty-four period versus fat, which is almost inert!

And, if that wasn't good enough, another group of researchers, Cowan and Gregory, reported in *Medicine & Science in Sports & Exercise,* assured us, *it's never too late.* This is what they found: ". . . menopausal status does not appear to lower a woman's ability to favorably alter her body composition and cardiorespiratory endurance through aerobic conditioning." Hooray! So, if you're one of those who thinks, "Why bother? Too late for me." Wrong. Wrong and double wrong!!

Losing weight is a basic numbers formula. . . and a pretty simple one at that. A pound of stored fat equals 3,500 calories. If you want to lose a pound of fat a week you decrease your energy intake (food) or increase your energy output (exercise) by 3,500. Simple. Well, we all know it's really not that simple. Exercise is hard and dieting is hard and it doesn't get any easier as we get older although it does become increasingly more important for health reasons.

I personally follow a very simple diet that is high in protein (fresh fish, lean meat, turkey, egg whites) high in fiber (lots of colorful fresh fruits and vegetables) and low in salt, fats, and sugars. Nothing fancy or complicated. If you have more than twenty pounds to lose or are suffering from any metabolic or health-related diet problems, I suggest you contact a registered dietician.

Here's the breakdown of how our bodies function:

1. Two thirds of our energy expenditure is used for our basal (or resting) metabolism, that is, the energy involved with maintaining body temperature and ionic gradients across cell membranes, contracting smooth muscle for cardiac and gastrointestinal function, and conducting other metabolic storage and mobilization processes. Fat-free mass (muscle) is the major contributor to the metabolic process.

2. Approximately 10% of our energy expenditure is dissipated through thermogenesis (the thermal effect of digesting food).

3. Activity and exercise accounts for the final 25% of the body's energy expenditure. The energy used for activity is related to body weight and the frequency, intensity, and duration of exercise.

This is good and important information to understand. As you can see, 25% of our body's weight management is within our complete control through proper exercise. That gives us a lot of power to make changes and a lot of motivation to choose wise and healthy options.

HOT FLASHES

Hot flashes are one of the major symptoms that occur in up to 75% of women in their menopausal years. Even though researchers are not certain why hot flashes occur (they suspect they are multifactorial), these vasomotor reactions to the volatility in your changing hormonal levels can result in loss of sleep and mood disturbances such as depression.

Dr. Burghart's findings reveal that, "For some women, regular exercise appears to be a promising alternative or adjunct to estrogen therapy. . . and may decrease the incidence and/or severity of hot flashes." Additionally, she cites a study that found ". . . both premenopausal women and postmenopausal women showed increased levels of estrogen after participating in an aerobic training program, and 55% of the postmenopausal women experienced a decrease in the severity of hot flashes."

BONE PROTECTION

The numbers are daunting: approximately 10 million Americans over the age of 50 have osteoporosis—thinning or loss of bone mass density. Another 34 million are at risk, suffering from low bone mass or osteopenia. Each year an estimated 1.5 million people suffer an osteoporotic-related fracture which can drastically and irretrievably reduce their quality of life and in some cases, lead to death. And who is at the greatest risk? Women, especially menopausal women. They are the most likely to develop osteoporosis and suffer osteoporotic-related fractures and mortality due to these events. It is estimated roughly four-in-ten Caucasian women aged fifty years or older in the United States will experience a hip, spine, or wrist fracture sometime during the remainder of their lives.

But there is good news and promising interventions. According to *The 2004 Surgeon General's Report on Bone Health and Osteoporosis,* "Physical activity is the only single therapy that can simultaneously improve muscle mass, muscle strength, balance and bone strength."

Along with good nutrition and supplemental calcium and vitamin D, physical activity is one of the most promising interventions to help keep your body strong and help prevent fractures from falls.

One other important point of information in the *Surgeon General's Report* was this: the impact of physical activity needs to be constant to maintain optimal bone health. So, if you stop participating in physical activity, your bones are no longer protected.

Again, what type of physical activities are the most beneficial for bone protection and maintenance? According to all the research, and as I wrote about earlier, you need to do exercises that are both *weight-bearing* (walking/hiking); and those that build and maintain muscle, *weight-resistance training*, which I will teach you how to do in the following strategies. Although exercise cannot absolutely reverse the impact of bone loss due to age and time, the evidence is strong that, as reported, ". . . it can modify and perhaps attenuate the process of deterioration in muscle and bone."

MOOD IMPROVEMENT

"So, what do you do to reduce stress in your life?" Sylvia asks me one day during her twice weekly training session. She is sixty-one and going through a difficult time, care-giving for her elderly father while taking care of her husband who recently suffered a mild stroke.

"Oh, I go for long walks and listen to tango music."

"That's your answer for everything isn't it? Exercise."

"No, not everything. If you asked how to make a lemon cake I'd give you a totally different answer. But yeah, for the most part, I think exercise really helps not only with your physical health, but with your mental health and well-being too."

I am not alone in my beliefs. Scientific research and clinical observations back me up on this. Exercise absolutely helps reduce stress and is often recommended as adjunctive therapy for women going through menopause.

In addition to hot flashes, weight gain, sleep disruption, and night sweats, women frequently report depression, mood change, fatigue, malaise, and irritability as symptoms of their menopausal transition.

In a paper entitled, "Women and Depression: Menopause," published by the University of Michigan Depression Center, the researchers recommend exercise as part of a complete program of therapy to treat menopausal depression. "Exercise helps treat depression by releasing the body's mood-elevating compounds, reducing the depression hormone cortisol . . . "

Other studies I have read on depression in menopausal women also draw a direct correlation between physical activity and mood improvement.

"Women of menopausal age who had the greatest increases in activity over a three-year period also reported the smallest increases in symptoms of stress and depression," reported researchers in an article appearing in the publication *Circulation*.

In an article published last year in the *Wall Street Journal*, Kevin Helliker writes, "A growing body of medical literature, including at least three 2005 studies, is showing that aerobic routines, as well as weight lifting are effective at combating depression. In addition to the famous 'runner's high' or endorphin surge that provides a temporary mood lift following a workout, the studies show that there is round-the-clock relief that sets in several weeks after the establishment of a regular exercise routine."

I created the following Anti-Aging Exercise Strategies and the Anti-Aging Workout Systems after years of experience as the clinical exercise specialist at UCLA and as a private health-fitness educator and practitioner. They are designed with one goal in mind: to give you the knowledge, tools, skills, and motivation to vault you into the next stage of your life—healthfully, beautifully, and happily.

"Legs" to Stand On
Movers and Shapers

Independence is for the very few; it is a privilege of the strong.

NIETZSCHE

I don't seem to have enough strength these days to pull myself up out of a chair," Lillian tells me. Lillian is sixty-eight and in good health, for the most part. She has been moderately physically active, gardening, walking with a walking group two or three times a week. But she has never done any kind of strength training.

"It's not for me. It's for young girls looking to wear bikinis to the beach. I'm not going to the beach and I'm certainly not going to be wearing any bikinis."

"Why not?" I tease. Then I go on to explain strength training is absolutely not just for "young girls."

One of the driving forces behind maintaining your physical strength is to maintain your freedom and independence throughout the aging process. This is a critical, life-defining issue for most menopausal women. They equate fear of growing older with "fear of growing weaker." The process of aging is by no means inevitably linked to the weakening of the body. Strength training is for all prideful people who want to age healthfully and beautifully.

LEGS TO STAND ON

Anti-Aging Strategy 3 is all about legs.

Your knee joint is the largest and most complicated joint in your entire body.

The muscle group in the front of your leg is called the quadriceps. As its name implies, it consists of four muscles: the rectus femoris, the vastus lateralis, the vastus intermedialis, and the vastus medialis. The rectus femoris, which is the muscle located in the middle of the front of your leg, is a two-jointed muscle, attaching from the lower part of your pelvic bone down to below your knee joint. The other three muscles in the group attach from the top of the femor (your leg bone) itself to the knee joint. It is this muscle group that allows you to do knee *extension.* Extending the knee would be the action you would be doing if you were sitting in a chair and trying on new shoes and you wanted to see how the shoe looked on your foot. You would extend your knee out in front of you so you could decide if you like it. (I do this when I try on my tango shoes. So far, I haven't found a pair I didn't like and buy.)

The muscle group located in the back of your leg is called the hamstrings and consists of three muscles: the semitendinosus, the semimembranosus and the biceps femoris. These muscles originate on the bottom of the pelvic bone and extend down around your knee joint. They are responsible for knee flexion, the opposite movement of knee extension. Your knee is in a flexed position when you are standing up and you bring your foot up toward your buttocks. (Not a good way to admire your new shoes.) The hamstring group is estimated to be 25% to 33% weaker than the quadriceps group. It is nicknamed the "running muscle" and it is the one you always hear about when a baseball player is running down to first base or a football player is running trying to catch a pass and suddenly they're down because of a hamstring pull. If you've lost your flexibility in bending forward to reach the floor with your hands, it is a result of tight hamstring muscles.

The back of your lower leg consists of two major muscles, the gastrocnemius and the soleus muscles, which are popularly referred to as your calf muscles. The "gastroc" starts on the lower part of the bone of your upper leg (femur) and attaches at your Achilles heel. The soleus originates on the backs of your two lower leg bones (tibia and fibula) and also attaches at your Achilles tendons. These two muscles working together are the ones that come into play when you are running, jumping, hopping or skipping. Ballet dancers who dance on pointe, for instance, have especially strong soleus muscles.

By protecting and preserving the muscles of your legs, you insure your physical strength and personal mobility, allowing you to continue to participate in, and enjoy activities that enrich your health, life, body, and spiritual well-being.

Body Preserving Exercises—Legs—Movers and Shapers

1   Leg Extensions Using Ankle Weights
2   Standing Hamstring Curls Using Ankle Weights
3   Standing Heel Raises Using Dumbbell
4   Plié Squats Against Exercise Ball
5   Inner Thigh Ball Squeezes
6   Side-Lying Inner Thigh Lifts Using Ankle Weights
7   Seated Leg Extensions
8   Hamstring Curls Using Ankle Weights Over Bench, Chair, or Ball
9   Machine Heel Raises
10 Machine Hamstring Curls

Equipment-Free Body Preserving Leg Exercises:

11 Lying Bent Knee Leg Lifts
12 Standing Hamstring Curls
13 Inner Thigh Squats (Froggies)
14 Heel Raises

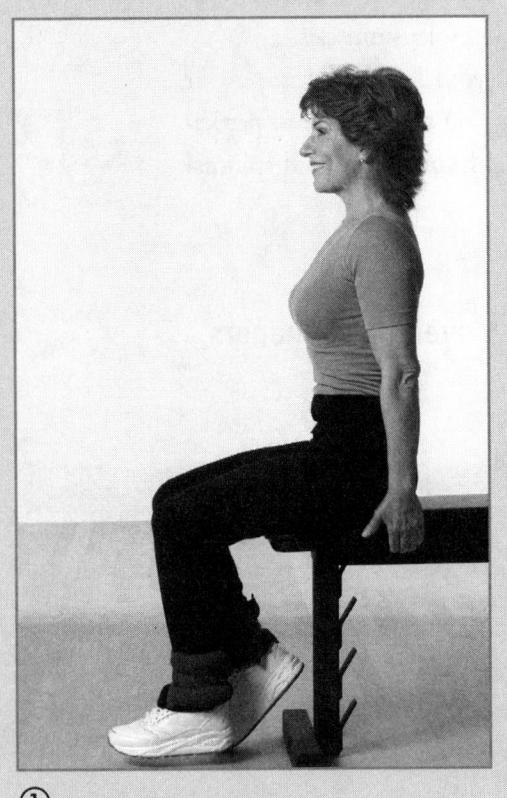

①

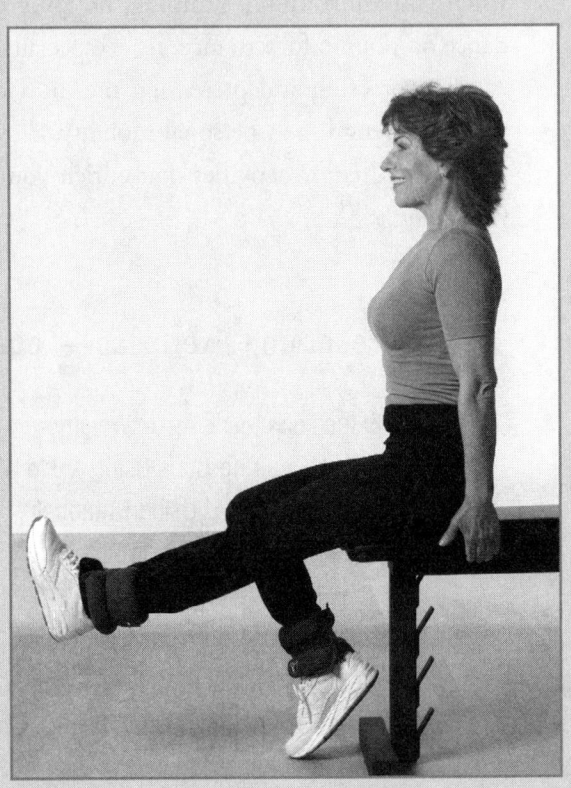

②

Leg Extensions Using Ankle Weights

EXECUTION

This is a great exercise you can not only do at the gym but also at home, in the office, or even while traveling. If you are not at the gym or using a workout bench, sit in a firm chair or on a piano bench. Strap on the ankle weights so they fit snugly and won't shift as you extend your leg. If the chair or bench you are sitting on doesn't have a back, sit up tall and straight, and contract the abs to help stabilize your trunk. It is fine to hold onto the side of the chair to give your body extra stability.

Lift one leg up, extend it so it is straight out in front of you while keeping a slight bend at the knee when it is parallel to the ground. Slowly return your leg to starting position but do not let it rest on the ground even for a moment, go immediately into your next repetition.

Muscles Working:
Front of Legs—
Quadriceps

Degree of Difficulty:
One Dumbbell

Equipment:
Ankle Weights

Body Position:
Seated

Form Watch:
As you lower your leg to starting position, do so slowly to feel the lengthening of the quadriceps muscles.

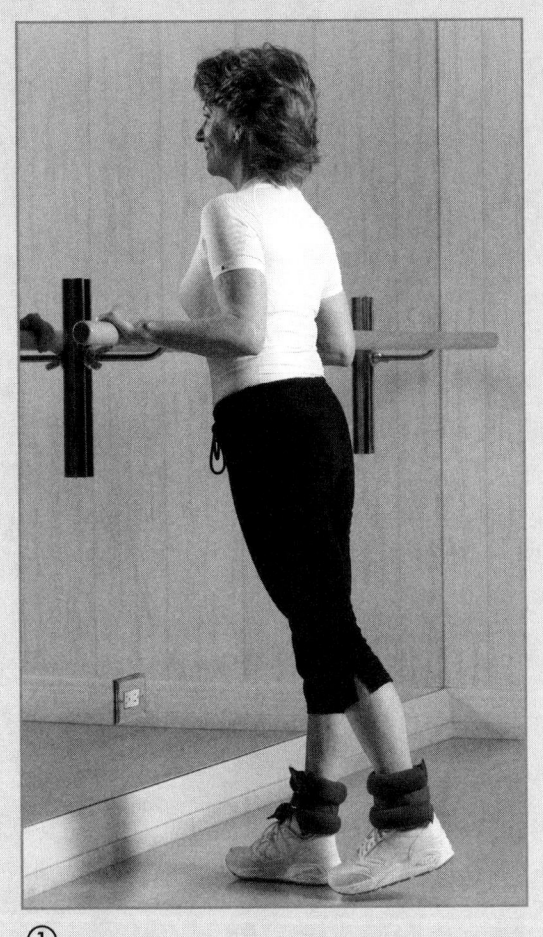

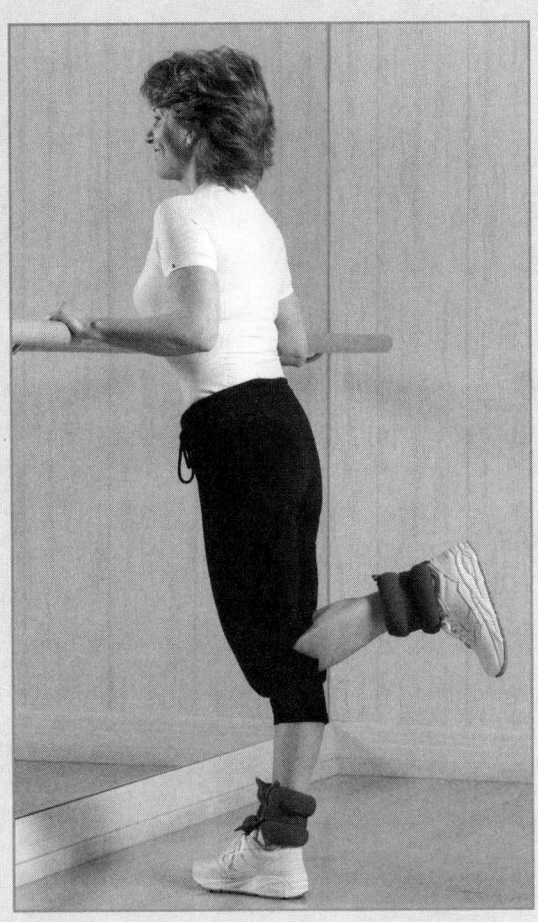

① ②

Standing Hamstring Curls Using Ankle Weights

EXECUTION

Strap the weights securely around your ankles. Place your hands against a wall or hold onto a ballet barre, counter, or the edge of a sturdy table. Your body should be at a slight angle, leaning forward. Contract your abdominals. Bring one foot off the floor— this is the start position. From there, bring your foot up and back toward your buttocks, squeezing the back muscles of the leg as you do. As you bring your foot down to starting position, do so slowly and feel the lengthening of the muscles.

Muscles Working:
Back of leg—
Hamstrings
(Semitendinous,
Semimembranosus,
Biceps Femoris)

Degree of Difficulty:
One Dumbbell

Body Position:
Standing

Form Watch:
Try and bring your foot as close to your buttocks as possible, contracting the leg muscles the entire time.

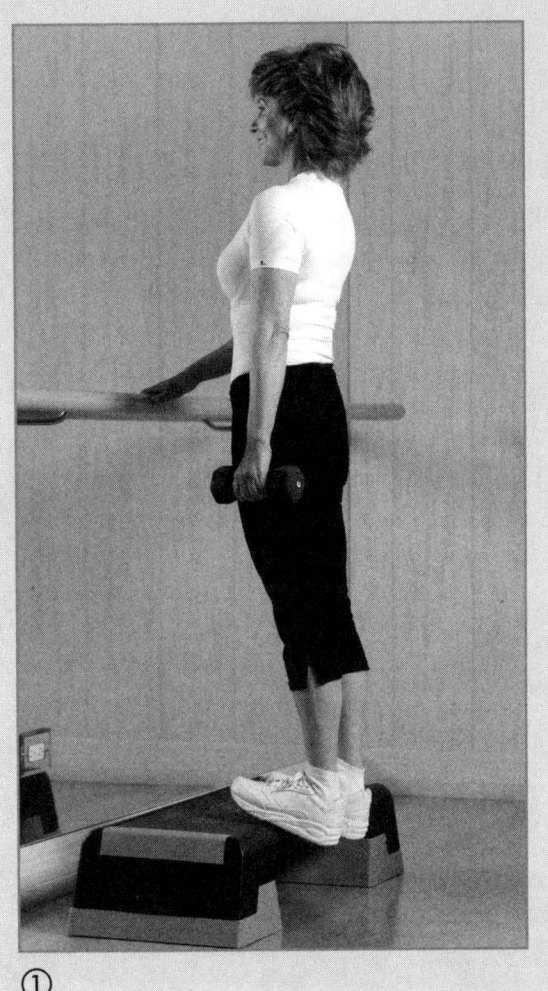

①

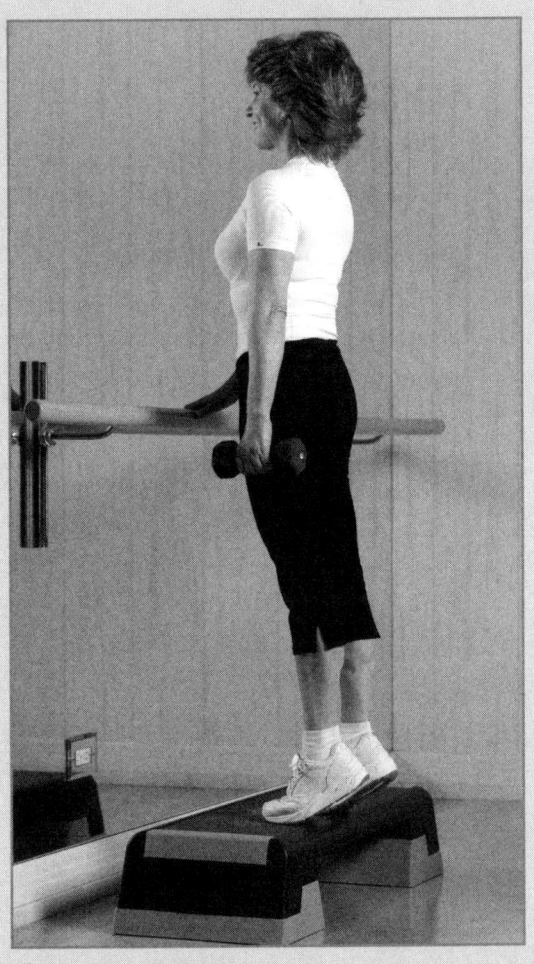

②

Standing Heel Raises Using Dumbbell

EXECUTION

Place your toes on the edge of a stair, step, or step stool so your heels are dropping below horizontal. Hold onto a ballet barre, counter, wall, or banister for support. In the hand not being used to supply support, place a dumbbell.

Standing tall, abdominals tightly contracted, slowly lift up your heels as far as you can and then immediately lower them as deeply as you. The reason you are standing on an elevated surface, is that it allows you to get a full range of motion in the ankle joint.

Muscles Working:
Calves
(Gastrocnemius,
Soleus)

Degree of Difficulty:
One Dumbbell

Equipment:
Dumbbell

Body Position:
Standing

Form Watch:
Keep your feet parallel to one another and try to get full extension both lifting and lowering your heels.

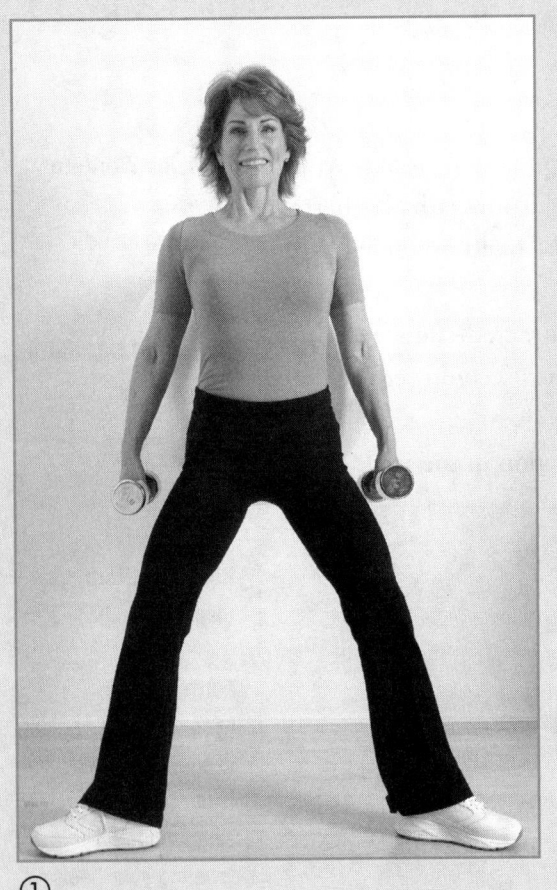

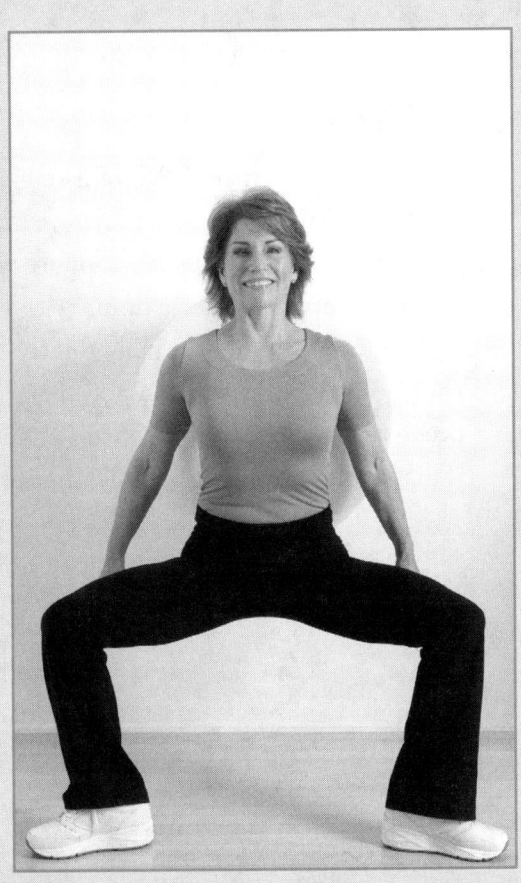

① ②

Plié Squats Against Exercise Ball

EXECUTION

If you do a plié leaning against an exercise ball, make sure you feel comfortable and secure using the ball. If you don't or if you don't own an exercise ball, you can also do them holding onto a ballet barre, countertop, or any other very stable object. If you are using a ball, place it against the wall so you can rest the middle of your back on it. As you drop into the plié, the ball rolls up your back.

Leaning against the exercise ball, place your feet shoulder-width apart with your toes pointed outward. In ballet, this is called second position.

Slowly drop into the plié position by bending your knees. Drop deeply enough to feel a contraction in the inner thigh muscles but don't go so far down that your knees go out over your toes.

Come back up and as you do make sure to squeeze the inner thighs.

This is a great way to work your inner thigh muscles either at the gym, at home, or even while traveling.

Muscles Working:
Inner Thigh Muscles (Adductors and Gracilis)

Degree of Difficulty:
One Dumbbell

Equipment:
Exercise Ball

Body Position:
Standing

Form Watch:
Keep your abdominals contracted, shoulders down, and spine straight.

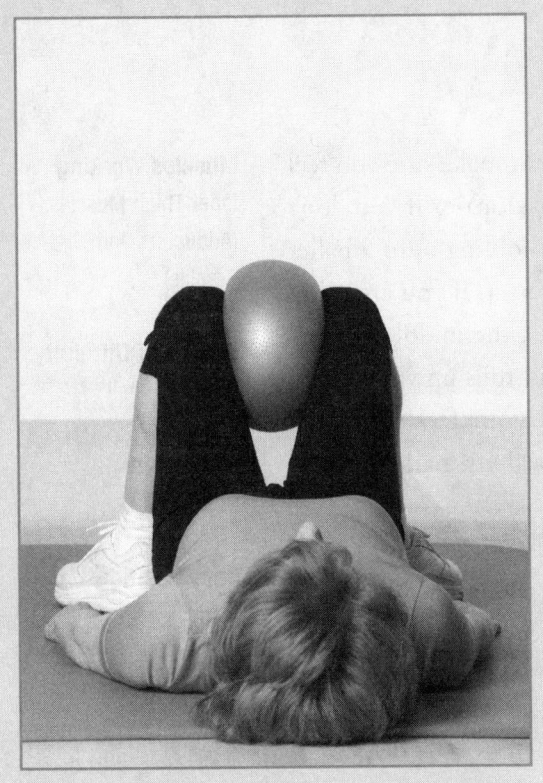

①

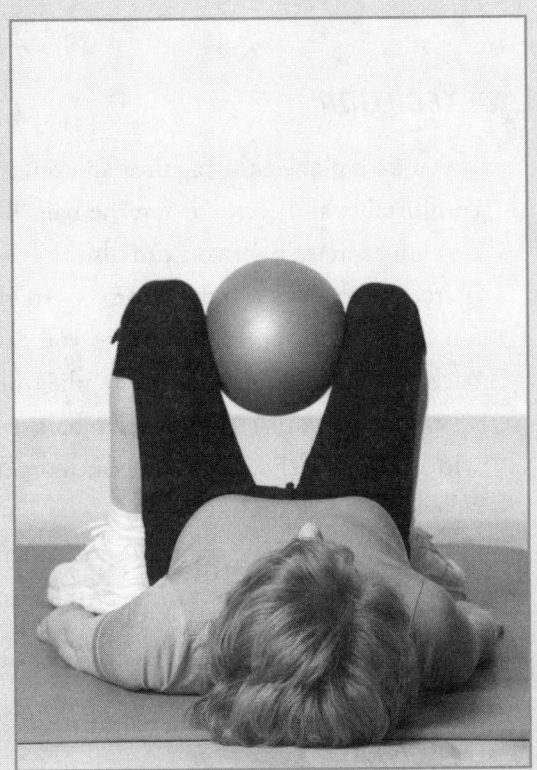

②

Inner Thigh Ball Squeezes

EXECUTION

For this exercise you will need a medium exercise ball about the size of a volleyball but softer so it can be squeezed. If you don't have a ball, you can simply roll up a towel so that it is about five inches thick and use that to supply the resistance.

Lie on the floor, knees bent and feet flat on the floor. Place the ball or towel securely between your thighs; once there, slowly press your knees together in small contractions so you feel your inner thighs tightening.

If you are sitting in a chair, place the ball or towel securely between your thighs and squeeze your knees together to contract the muscles.

Muscles Working:
Inner Thighs—
Adductor Longus,
Gracilis

Degree of Difficulty:
One Dumbbell

Equipment:
Small Exercise Ball

Body Position:
Lying on floor or
seated in a chair

Form Watch:
If you are doing this exercise seated in a chair, make sure your abdominals are contracted and you are sitting up straight with good posture.

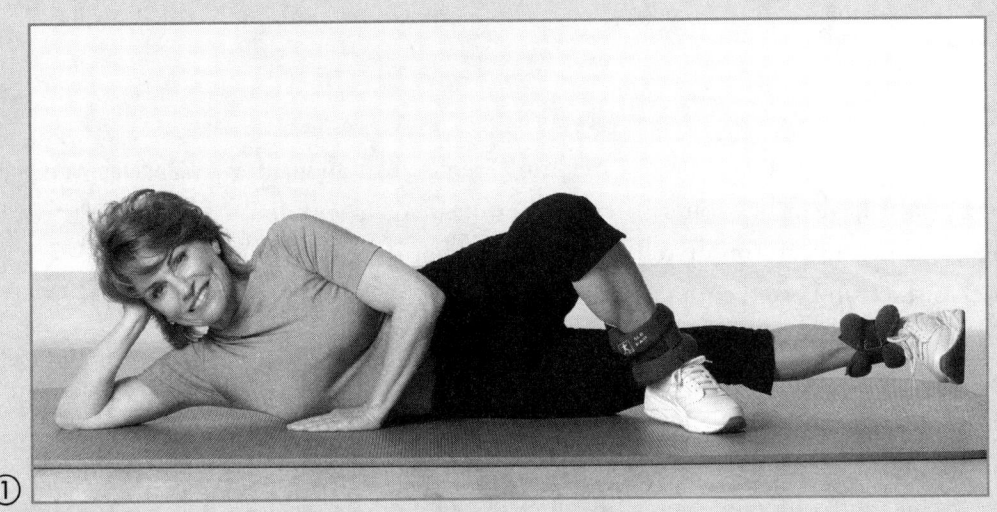

①

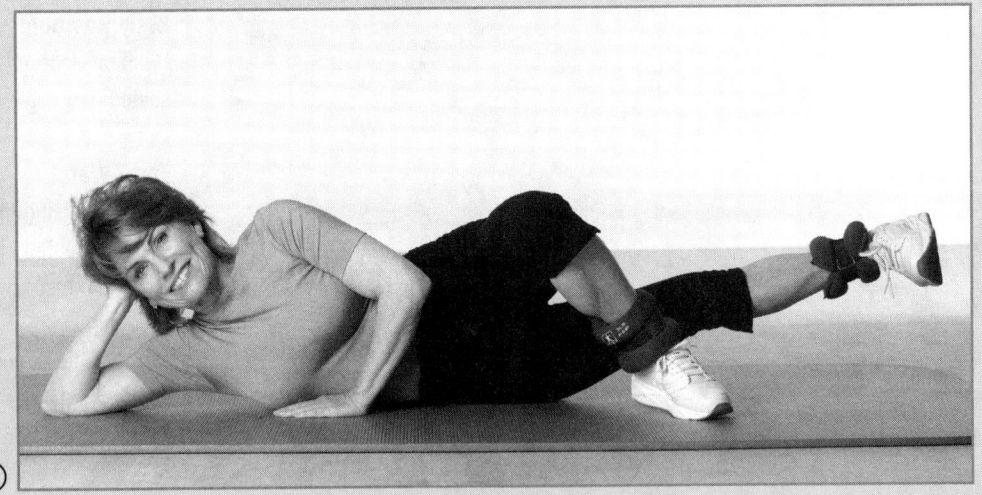

②

Side-Lying Inner Thigh Lifts Using Ankle Weights

EXECUTION

Lying on your side, place your head either in your hand to protect your neck or rest it on your outstretched arm, whatever is most comfortable for you. Take your top leg and bring it over your bottom leg and place the foot of that leg on the floor, creating a "bridge" over the bottom leg. Wrap an ankle weight around the bottom leg, which is straight out; the foot of the bottom leg is flexed hard enough so you feel a tightening muscle of the inner thigh.

Lift the bottom leg up about two inches off the ground. This is your starting position. From there lift the leg as far up as you can, which might only be twelve inches. It is not a big range of motion. Immediately return your leg to the starting position without touching the floor. This is a continuous motion exercise and the leg should not touch the floor until all repetitions are completed.

Muscles Working:
Inner Thigh Muscles (Adductors and Gracilis)

Degree of Difficulty:
One Dumbbell

Equipment:
Ankle Weights

Body Position:
Lying on the floor

Form Watch:
Maintain your body position without rocking back and forth and keep your abdominals contracted.

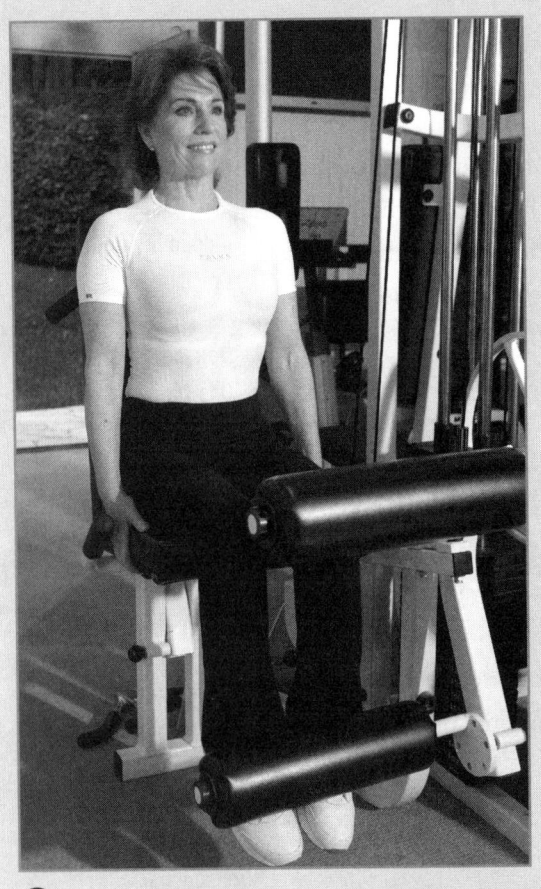

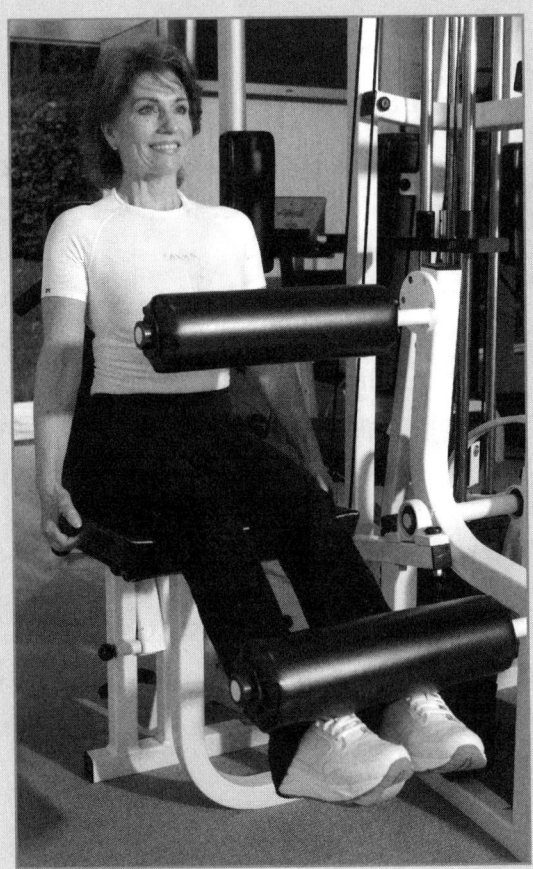

① ②

Seated Leg Extensions

EXECUTION

Adjust your position on the machine so your back is pressed firmly against the seat to protect your spine and lower back. Even though you are seated, make sure your abdominal muscles are contracted. Don't slouch! Place the roller bar so it rests just around your ankles. You don't want it to be too far down on your foot. Many machines have places to grip with your hands to stabilize your body or you can hold onto the seat with your hands for support.

Extend your legs out in front of you so they are almost parallel to the floor but do not extend them so they are completely straight and locking out your knees. You want to keep a slight bend in the knee at all times.

As you bring your legs back down to start position, move slowly contracting the muscles through the full range of motion. If you place your hand onto your thigh, you will feel the muscle tightening so you know it is working!

Muscles Working:
Front of Legs
(Quadriceps)

Degree of Difficulty:
Two Dumbbells

Equipment:
Leg Extension
Machine

Body Position:
Seated

Form Watch:
Sit up straight in the seat and watch your posture.

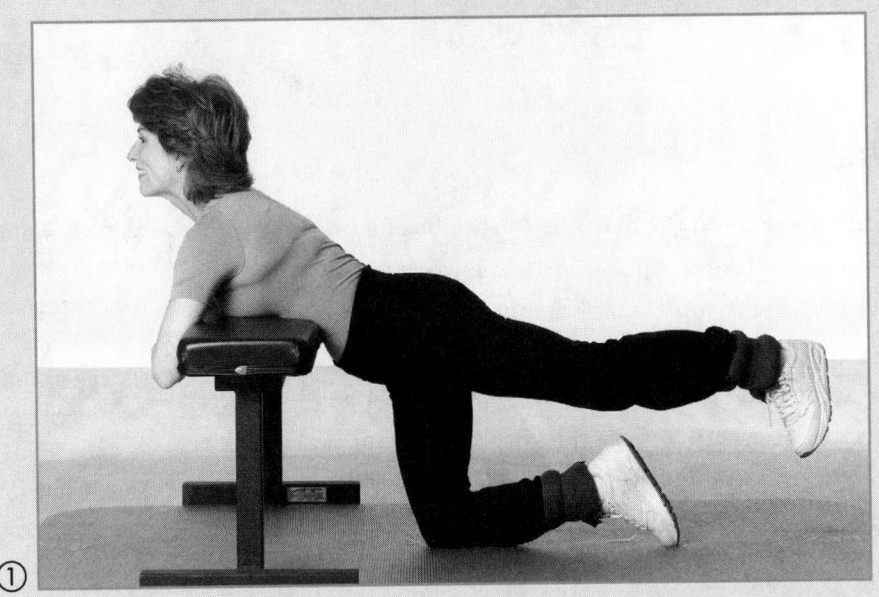

①

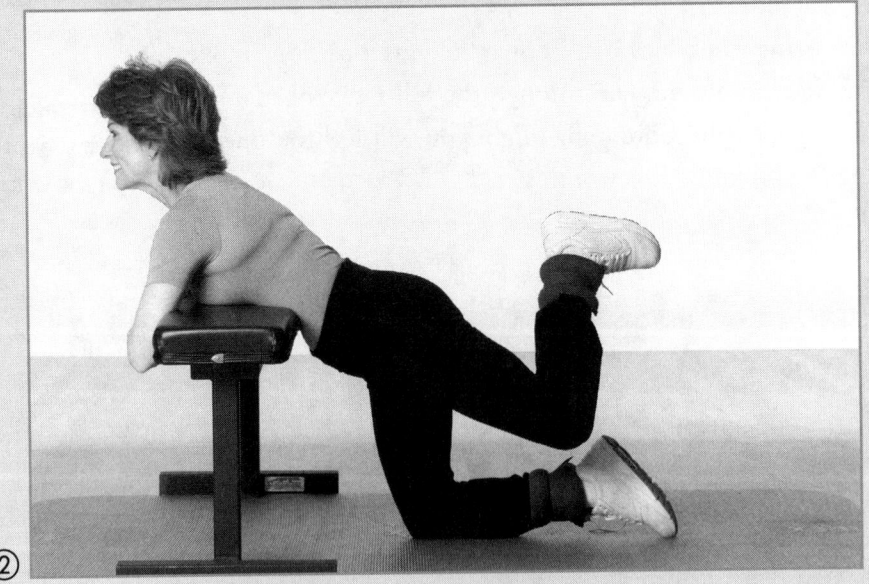

②

Hamstring Curls Using Ankle Weights Over Bench, Chair, or Ball

EXECUTION

Place your torso so you're resting comfortably over a ball, chair, or a bench. You can brace your upper body by holding onto the edge of the bench. If using a ball, place it up against a wall or a bench so it is stable.

Lift one leg off the floor straight out behind you. When it is parallel to the ground, slowly curl your foot towards your buttocks. Release slowly to starting position (leg out straight behind you) and repeat curl movement again towards your buttocks. Repeat with the other leg.

Muscles Working:
Back of Leg—
Hamstrings
(Semitendinous,
Semimembranosus,
Biceps Femoris)

Degree of Difficulty:
Two Dumbbells

Equipment:
Ankle Weights, Bench,
Chair, or Ball

Body Position:
Upper body resting
over a bench, chair,
or ball

Form Watch:
Keep your core
muscles, abs,
contracted the entire
time, which will help
stabilize your body
and help protect your
lower back.

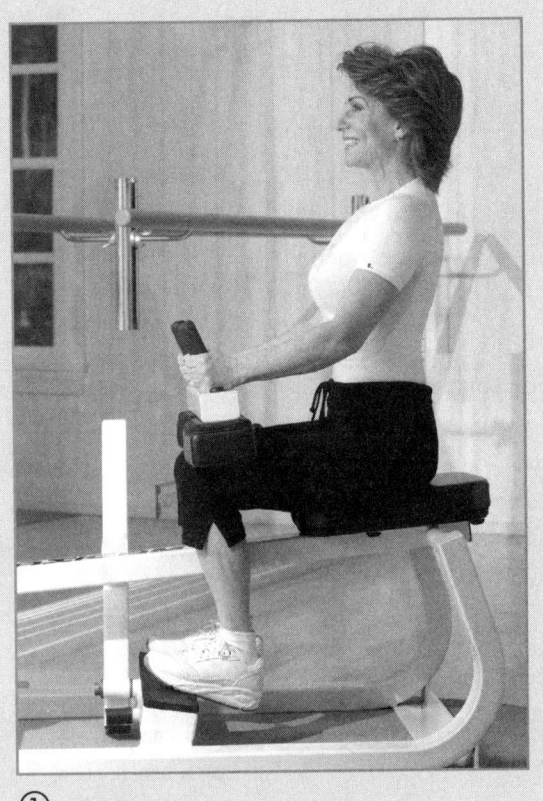
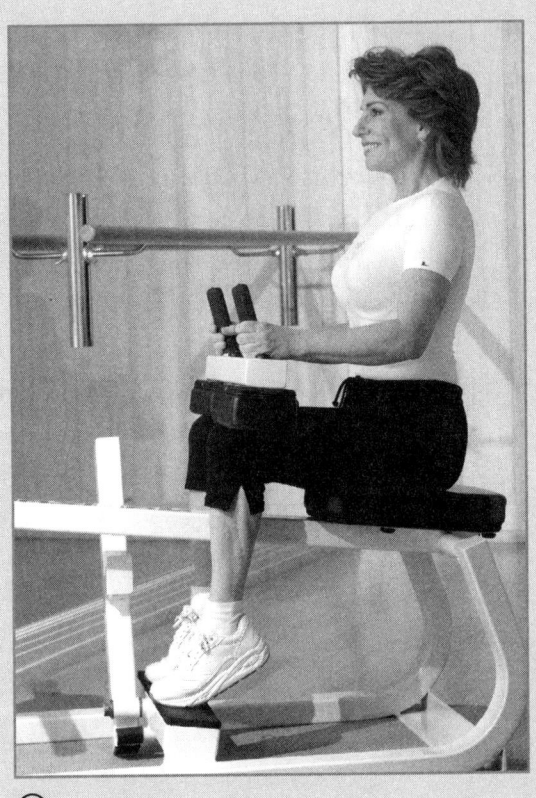

① ②

Machine Heel Raises

EXECUTION

There are two different style of machines designed for doing heel raises. One is a seated machine, often times called a "donkey press" and the other is one on which you stand upright (there are variations of these in the gym, but for the most part, these two styles are the basic designs).

    If you are using the seated "donkey press" sit comfortably on the machine and place your toes on the platform so your heels are below the platform. Then you lift your heels up as far as you can and then slowly lower them as deeply as possible until you feel a strong pull in back of your legs and into your heel cords.

Muscles Working:
Back of Lower Legs—
Calf Muscles
(Gastrocnemius,
Soleus)

Degree of Difficulty:
Two Dumbbells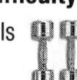

Equipment:
Machine

Body Position:
Seated or Standing

Form Watch:
Don't lean over the machine. Sit up straight and keep abdominals contracted.

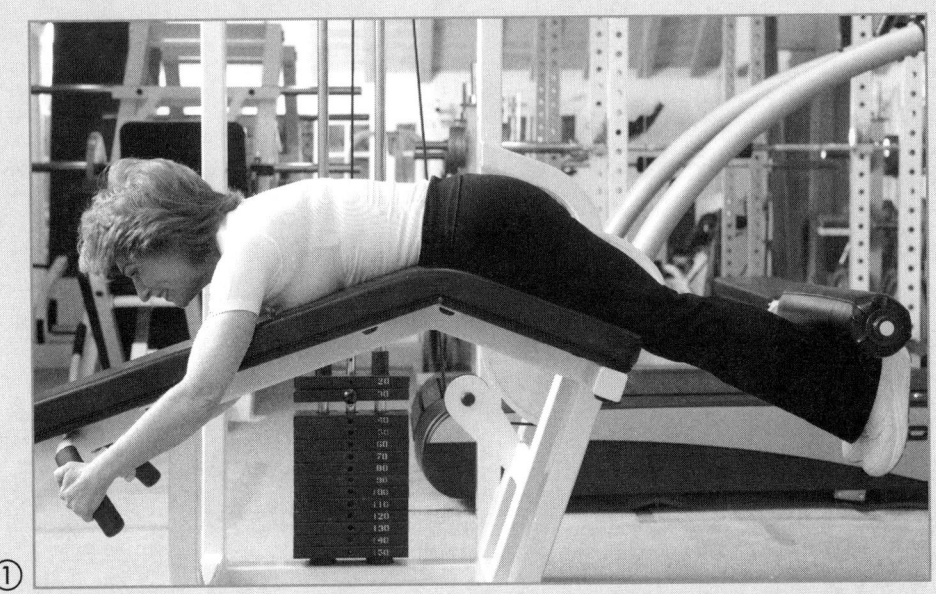

①

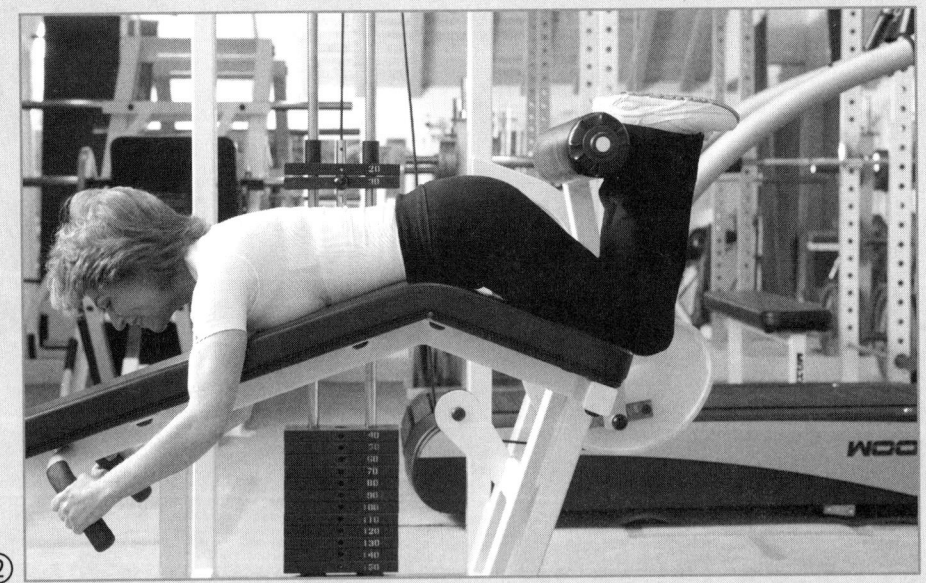

②

Machine Hamstring Curls

EXECUTION

Lying comfortably on your stomach, position yourself on the machine so that the backs of your ankles are hooked under the foot bar. You can hold onto the sides of the machine with your hands for extra support.

In this position, slowly lift the foot bar up toward your buttocks. As you curl your legs up, squeeze the muscles so you feel a strong contraction in the back of your upper legs.

As you lower the foot bar to starting position, do not let it simply fall back, but resist strongly against the pull of gravity by using the back leg muscles to provide the force of resistance. You will feel a lengthening of the muscles as you lower the foot bar back to starting position.

Muscles Working:
Back of Leg—
Hamstrings
(Semitendinous,
Semimembranosus,
Biceps Femoris)

Degree of Difficulty:
Three Dumbbells

Equipment:
Leg Curl Machine

Body Position:
Lying on Machine

Form Watch:
Don't rush the movement. Try and take the same amount of time doing the upward curl as you do to release the foot bar to the starting position. Make sure your hips do not lift off the machine.

Lying Bent Knee Leg Lifts

Muscles Working:
Front of Leg—
Quadriceps

Degree of Difficulty:
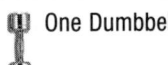 One Dumbbell

Equipment:
None Required

Body Position:
Lying

Form Watch:
Even though this is a
floor exercise, make
sure you keep your
abdominal muscles
contracted the
entire time.

EXECUTION

Lying on your back on the floor, your knees are bent and your feet are flat on the floor in front of you about twelve to fourteen inches, creating the space of a triangle between your feet and your body. Abdominals are contracted and your neck and shoulders are relaxed. Without moving your knee from its bent position, lift your foot up off the ground slowly bringing your knee toward your chest. Bring your leg up as far as possible and then slowly bring it back down toward the floor but do not rest it on the floor. This is a continuous movement until you've completed all repetitions.

Standing Hamstring Curls

EXECUTION

Stand up tall, holding onto a ledge or countertop, or placing your hands flat against a wall for support. If you are using a wall for support, place your hands shoulder-width apart and your feet about two feet from the wall. Contract your abdominal muscles. Make certain your hips are parallel to one another, so one does not come out in front of the other. Keep shoulders and neck relaxed.

Lift one foot off the ground and slowly curl the heel of the foot back toward your buttocks. As you bring your foot up, contract the muscles in the back of your leg. As you release, do so slowly, feeling the muscles lengthening as your bring your foot back down to starting position. This is a continuous action exercise. Do not let the foot rest on the floor but begin the next repetition immediately. (See photo on page 38 as an example of proper form and technique for this exercise.)

Muscles Working:
Back of leg—
Hamstrings
(Semitendinous,
Semimembranosus,
Biceps Femoris)

Degree of Difficulty:
One dumbbell

Equipment:
None Required

Body Position:
Standing

Form Watch:
Try and bring your foot as close to your buttocks as possible.

Inner Thigh Squats (Froggies)

Muscles Working:
Inner Thigh Muscles
(Adductors and
Gracilis)

Degree of Difficulty:
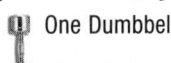 One Dumbbell

Equipment:
None Required

Body Position:
Lying on the floor

Form Watch:
Concentrate on
squeezing the
muscles of the inner
thighs, especially as
you lift them back to
starting position.

EXECUTION

This is a wonderful exercise that you can do either at home or in the gym, almost anywhere (except in a restaurant or driving a car!). Lie on your back in a comfortable position. Lift your legs up straight above you. Turn your feet so your toes and heels from both feet are touching, creating a diamond-like space between your legs. Now bring your feet down toward your pelvic area, which brings both knees out to either side. Now bring your legs up to starting, straight-legged position.

Heel Raises

EXECUTION

Stand facing the back of a sturdy chair, countertop, or table. Place a hand on the chair for balance. You can also do this on a step in your house or on a stairwell or steps outside your house as long as there is a rail or something you can hold onto for balance. If standing on a step or stair, you will be able to get a fuller range of motion by placing your toes as close to the edge as possible. Stand tall, contract your abdominals, and keep your shoulders and neck relaxed. Whether you are standing on a step or stair or on the ground, lift your heels up as high as you can. You will feel a stretch in the back of your legs. Slowly drop your heels down as deeply as possible. If you are standing on a step or a stair you will be able to drop your heels past the horizontal position. Keep a slight bend in your knees at all times. (See photo on page 40 as an example of proper form and technique for this exercise.)

Muscles Working:
Back of Lower Legs—
Calf Muscles
(Gastrocnemius,
Soleus)

Degree of Difficulty:
One Dumbbell

Equipment:
None Required

Body Position:
Standing

Form Watch:
Keep your abdominal muscles contracted and maintain good posture by standing tall, shoulders back, head in alignment with your spine.

Behind the Scenes:
"Hip" and "Buttocks"
Smoothers and Lifters

It is easy to live for others: everybody does. I call on you to live for yourselves.

EMERSON

My friend Tina turned to me in the dressing room while she was trying on a pair of denim jeans one day and said, "I know your face is supposed to fall, but your butt, too? This is most unfair."

"Most unfair," I agreed. "But not inevitable. You're losing muscle," I told her.

"In my butt?"

"Yes, in your butt, all over."

Tina is forty-eight and of normal weight. She works as an accountant, so she spends a lot of time behind a desk.

"I know I sit a lot in front of the computer crunching numbers. But I play tennis twice a week. Shouldn't that help preserve my behind?"

"It might help a little, but in order to really give your butt a boost, you have to be doing some strength training exercises that specifically target your glutes."

"My what?"

"Your glutes . . . gluteals . . . the muscle of the buttocks. They help power you forward. They are the primary muscles activated in walking, climbing stairs, bending, and lifting. The stronger this muscle group, the stronger your entire body feels."

"If I do these "glute" exercises, will my tennis game improve?"

"It's a good possibility. You'll move with increased force and confidence," I assured her. I'd never seen her play tennis and didn't want to make any promises I could not keep, but this I could guarantee: "You'll look a lot better in your in jeans."

Like most women, Tina didn't fully realize she was losing muscle throughout the aging process and how important a weight-training program was to preserving not only her strength, but her overall health.

"A better butt and a better game of tennis. Lead the way."

Leading the way is exactly what the action of the gluteal muscle group does. The three major muscles that comprise this group, mostly referred to as your buttocks, are the gluteus maximus, gluteus medius, and the gluteus minimus. The gluteus maximus is strongly engaged when you run, jump, hop, and skip, or walk with very aggressive, long strides. The gluteus medius and gluteus minimus are important muscles used in normal walking, so that as your weight shifts from side to side your hips stay in alignment.

The following exercises are what I like to call butt blasters and beautifiers. They are also responsible for giving you functional strength and mobility, freedom and flexibility of movement. No "buts" about it.

Body Preserving Exercises—Hip and Buttocks Smoothers and Lifters

1 Ball Squats
2 Dumbbell Squats
3 Single Leg Lunges with Resistance Ball
4 Side-Lying Leg Lifts Using Exercise Band
5 Step-Ups Using Body Bar or Dumbbells
6 Reverse Lunges Using Ankle Weights
7 Squats on Smith Machine

Equipment-Free Body Preserving Hip and Buttocks Exercises:

8 Standing Side Leg Lifts
9 Standing Rear Leg Lifts
10 Stationary Lunges
11 Reverse Lunges
12 Sit Downs

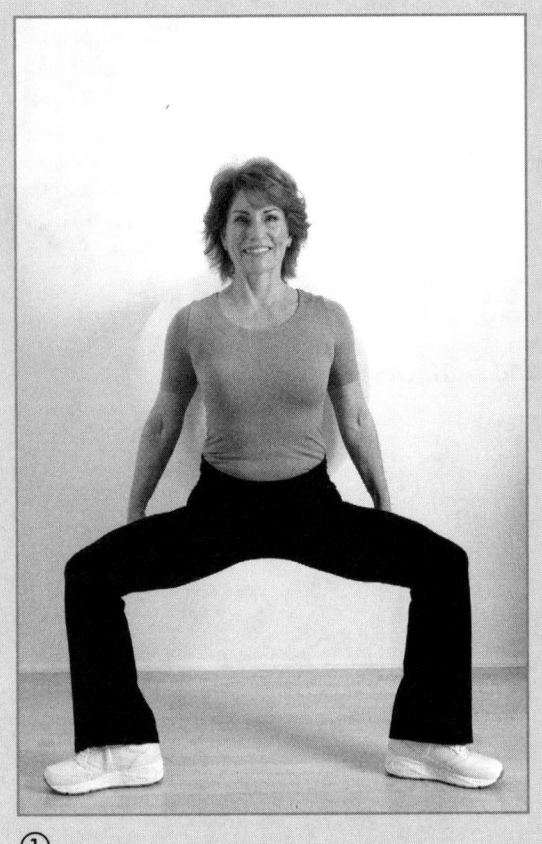

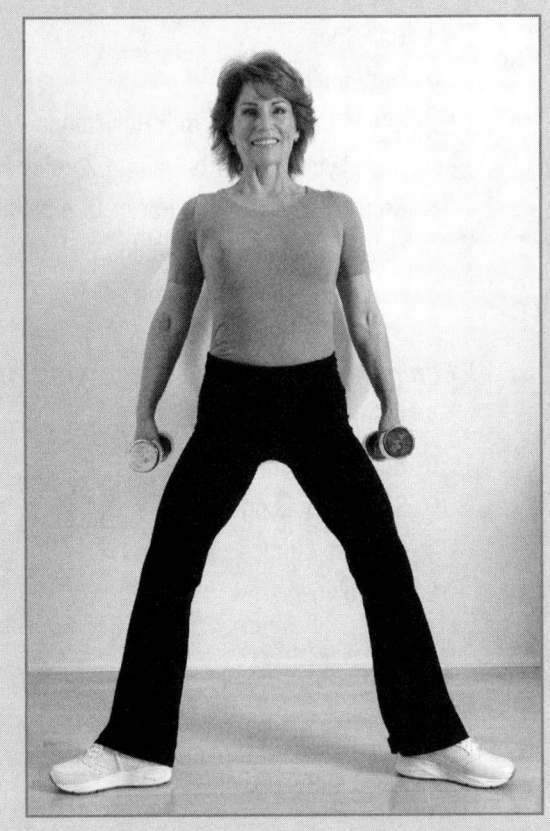

① ②

Ball Squats

EXECUTION

This is an exercise that you can do at home as well as in the gym.

Place the ball on a wall where there is room enough for it to roll up and down as you perform the squat. Place the ball so it rests in the middle of your back. With your back resting on the ball, place both your feet on the floor in front of you far enough from your body to allow yourself to drop down into the squat position. If you are comfortable using the ball and want to add some resistance, you can hold dumbbells in either hand. Before you drop into the squat, contract your abdominals tightly, which will help stabilize you on the ball.

As you drop down, make certain your knees do not go out over your toes. When your thighs are parallel to the ground, come back up slowly to starting position, keeping your buttocks muscles contracted the entire time.

Muscles Working:
Buttocks and Front of Legs— Gluteals and Quadriceps

Degree of Difficulty:
One Dumbbell

Equipment:
Exercise Ball and Dumbbells (optional)

Body Position:
Standing

Form Watch:
The ball should align with your spine as you drop into the squat.

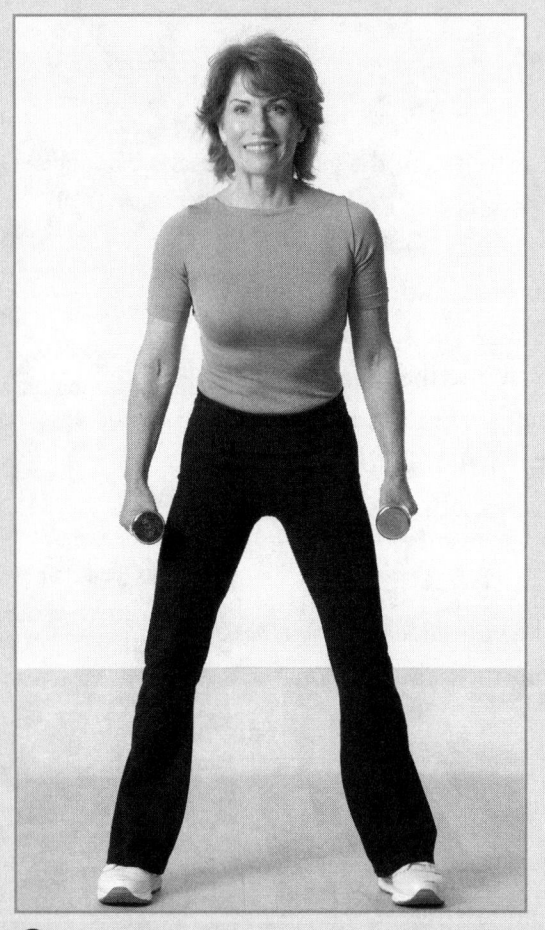

①

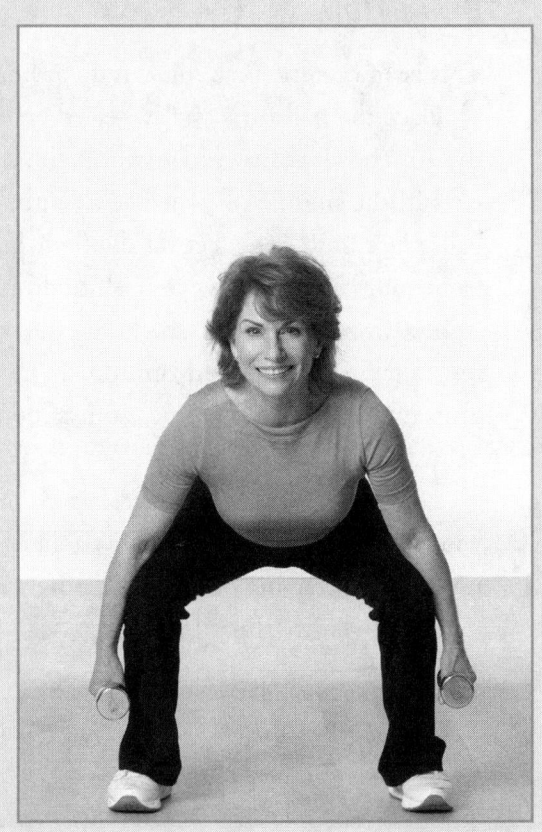

②

Dumbbell Squats

EXECUTION

Stand with your feet slightly wider than hip distance apart. Place a dumbbell in each hand. Your fingertips are facing toward your thighs. Contract your abdominals and stand tall. Feet are parallel to one another.

Bend your knees and lower your body as if you were going to sit in a very low chair. Your torso will be angled slightly forward to accommodate the move as you bend your knees into a 90-degree angle. You will want to maintain a natural arch in the lower back. Stay in the squat position for about two to three seconds, then come up slowly by straightening your knees till you are standing in full upright position.

Muscles Working:
Buttocks—
Gluteals and
Quadriceps

Degree of Difficulty:
Two Dumbbells

Equipment:
Dumbbells

Body Position:
Standing

Form Watch:
Do not let your knees come out over your toes when you are in the full squat position.

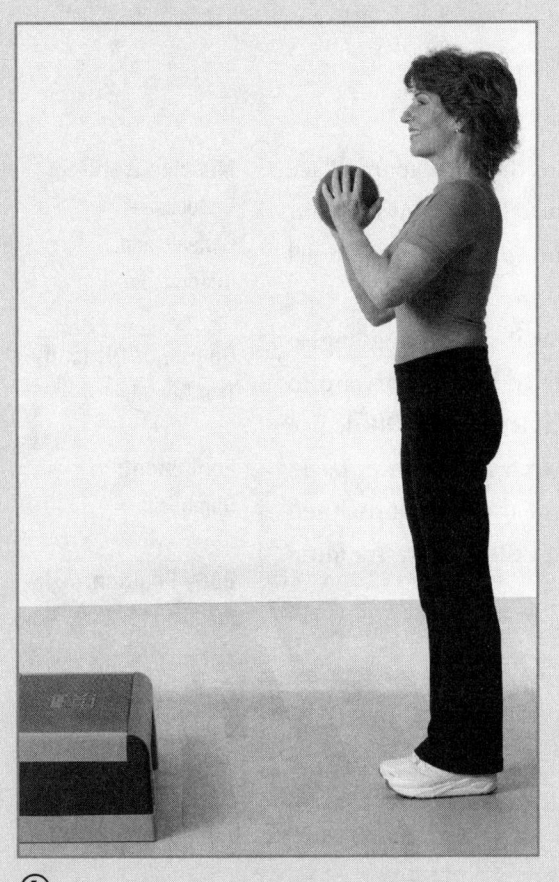

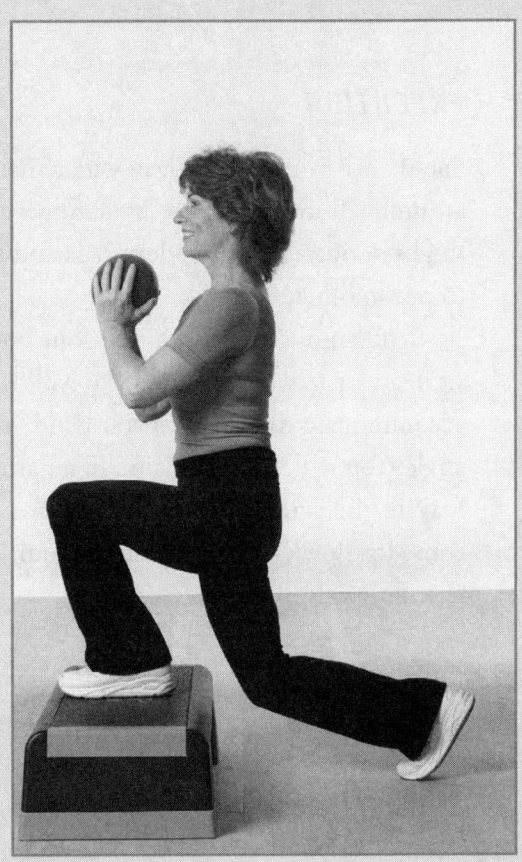

Single Leg Lunges with Resistance Ball

EXECUTION

Lunges are one of the best exercises you can do to firm and strengthen your buttocks. However, a word of caution: if you have bad knees, do not do these exercises. You can hold a weighted exercise ball or dumbbells in your hands to add some resistance, or lunge equipment free, if you prefer.

Standing tall with your feet together, abs contracted, spine straight, step forward with one leg, bending the front knee as you move ahead. The back leg bends automatically as you execute this forward motion. You will feel a contraction in both the buttocks muscles and on the top of the thigh of the forward lunging leg.

Step back into start position and lunge forward again with the same leg to continue the series of repetition.

If you feel you can't keep your balance, it is perfectly fine to do the forward lunge holding onto a countertop or any sturdy piece of furniture with one hand while holding a dumbbell in the other for added resistance.

Muscles Working:
Buttocks and Front of Legs—
Gluteals and Quadriceps

Degree of Difficulty:
Two Dumbbells

Equipment:
Step Platform and Weighted Exercise Ball (Optional: A Dumbbell)

Body Position:
Standing

Form Watch:
Make sure your knee does not go out beyond your toe.

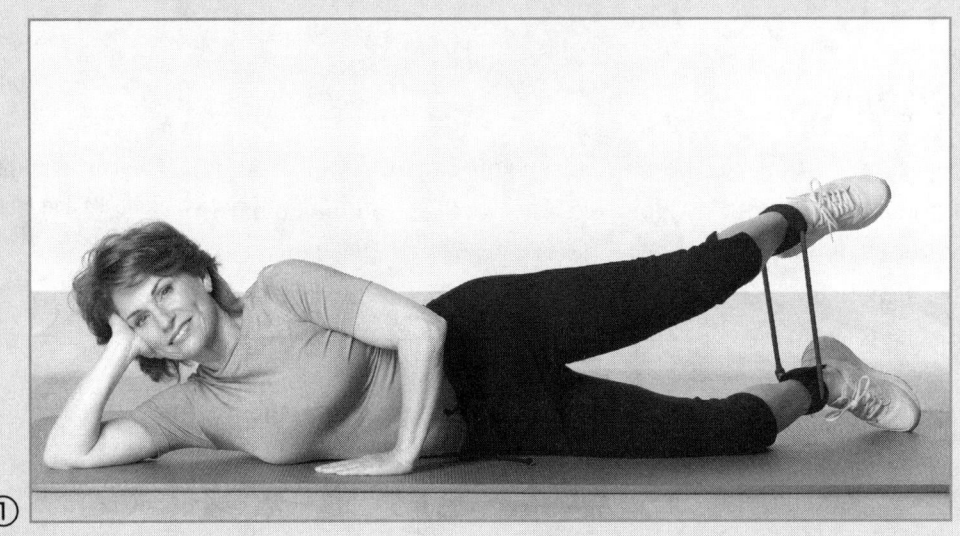

①

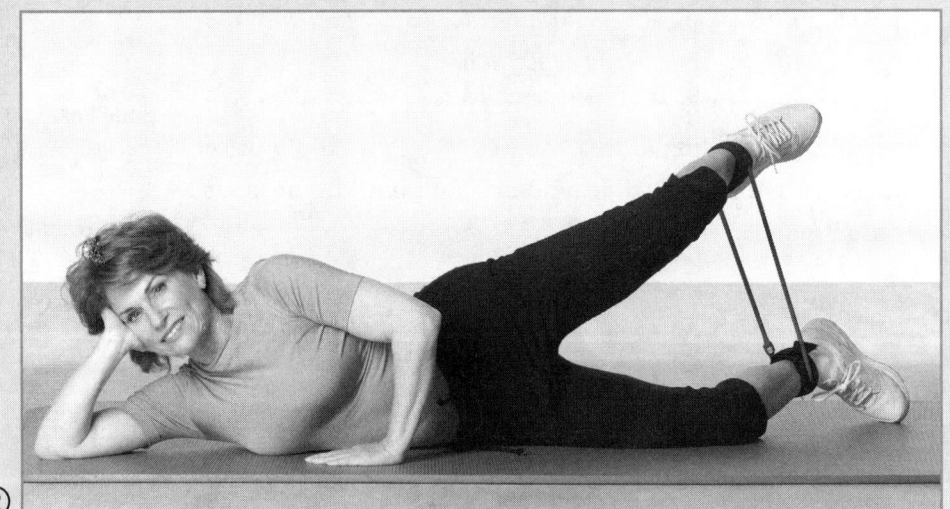

②

Side-Lying Leg Lifts Using Exercise Band

EXECUTION

Lying on your side, place your head either in your hand to protect your neck or rest it on your outstretched arm, whatever is most comfortable for you. Place your legs so they are in a straight line with your torso. Your knees have a slight bend in them and they are parallel to one another. Lift your top leg up enough so that the exercise band is taut. Starting from this position, lift your working leg up so the band is fully expanded and you feel a strong contraction on the side of your legs and buttocks.

Muscles Working:
Buttocks (Gluteus Medius)

Degree of Difficulty:
Two Dumbbells

Equipment:
Exercise Band

Body Position:
Lying

Form Watch:
Place your legs with enough distance between them that the exercise band never goes slack.

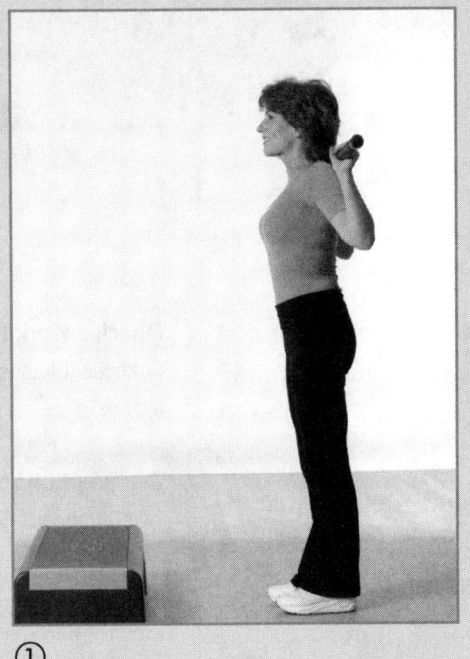

①

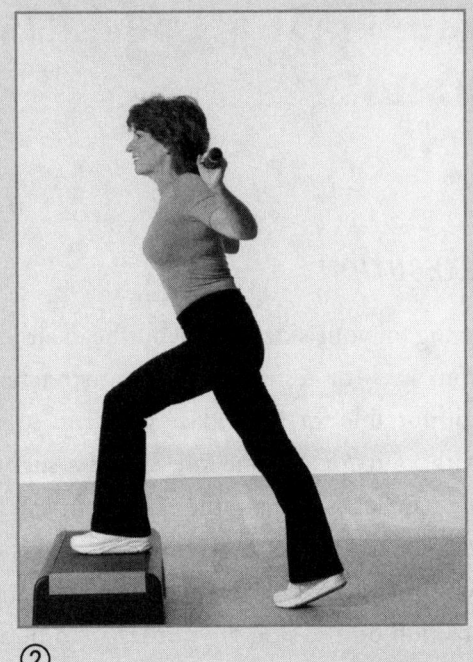

②

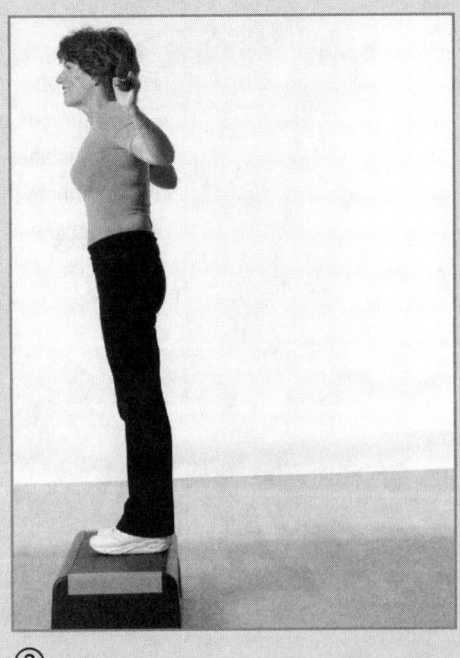

③

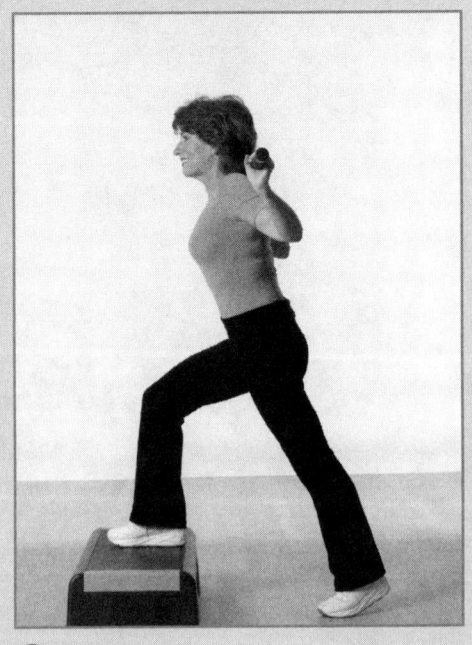

④

Step-Ups Using Body Bar or Dumbbells

EXECUTION

Place the step platform in front of you so you have plenty of room to step up on to it and back off of it.

If you are holding dumbbells, place them firmly in your hands with your arms hanging down by the sides of your legs. If you are using a body bar, place it so it is evenly distributed along the top on your shoulders. You can also hold it in front of you, if you prefer.

With your abdominals tightly contracted and spine straight, step onto the platform with one foot then immediately step up with the other foot. Step backward off the platform with the foot you first stepped on with, followed by the second foot.

Steps-Up are done in a continuous motion until you complete your repetitions.

If you are doing these in a gym or fitness facility, you can also use a barbell, which you would place above your shoulders.

The higher the platform you are stepping on, the more difficult the exercise. So if you are new to this exercise, start on a lower platform.

Muscles Working:
Buttocks and Front of Legs—
Gluteals and Quadriceps

Degree of Difficulty:
Two Dumbbells

Equipment:
Step Platform, Body Bar or Dumbbells

Body Position:
Standing

Form Watch:
Make sure you are standing up straight, keeping your shoulders back and abdominals contracted.

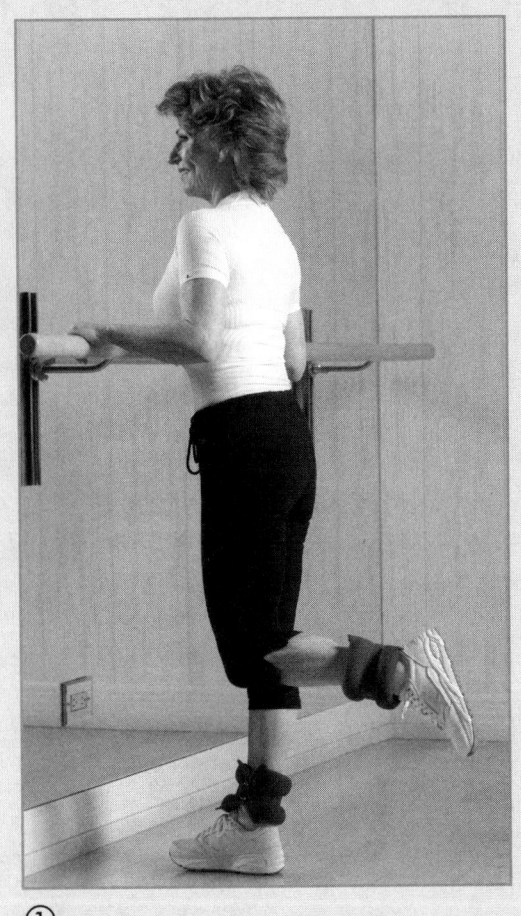

①

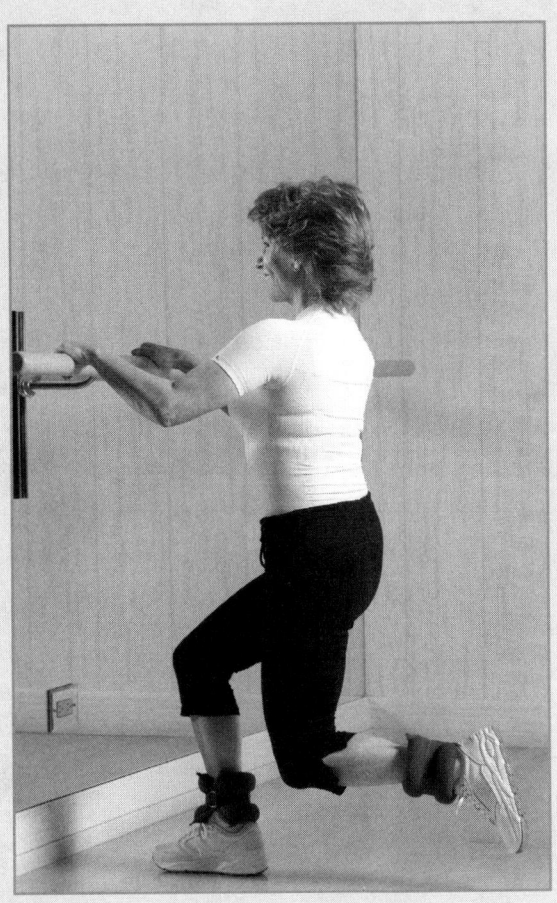

②

Reverse Lunges Using Ankle Weights

EXECUTION

Holding onto a stationary object—a ballet barre, door handle, sturdy table or countertop—stand straight with your abdominals contracted. Bring one leg behind you bending the knee so your leg is at a 90-degree angle to your body. Your torso should remain tall, back straight, chest open, and head high.

From starting position, you lunge backward by bending the knee of the leg you are standing on into a 90-degree angle without letting your toes come out over your knee. Try and bring your bent back leg so it is parallel to the ground while contracting the glute muscles the entire time. Hold the lunge for about three seconds and return to starting position.

Muscles Working:
Buttocks and Front of Legs—
Gluteals and Quadriceps

Degree of Difficulty:
Three Dumbbells

Equipment:
Ankle Weights

Body Position:
Standing

Form Watch:
Stand tall the entire time without letting your torso fall forward or backward.

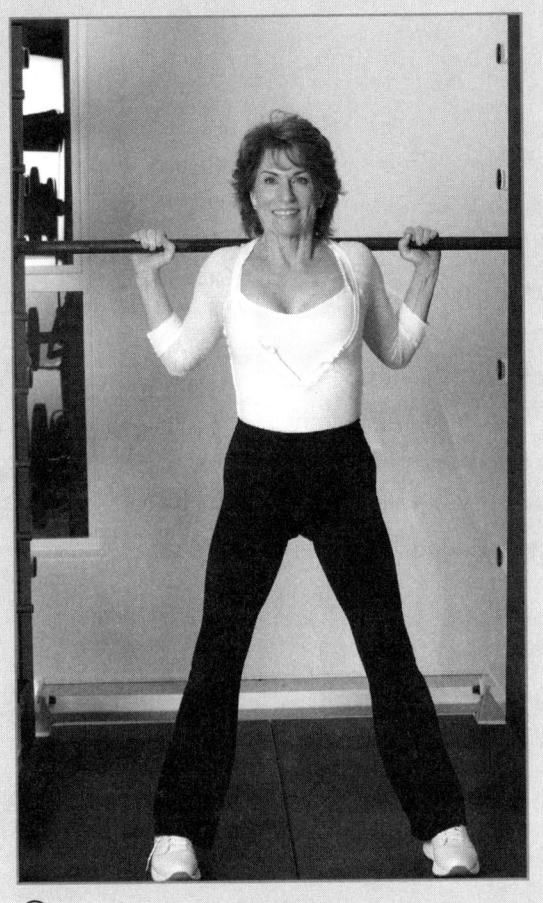

①

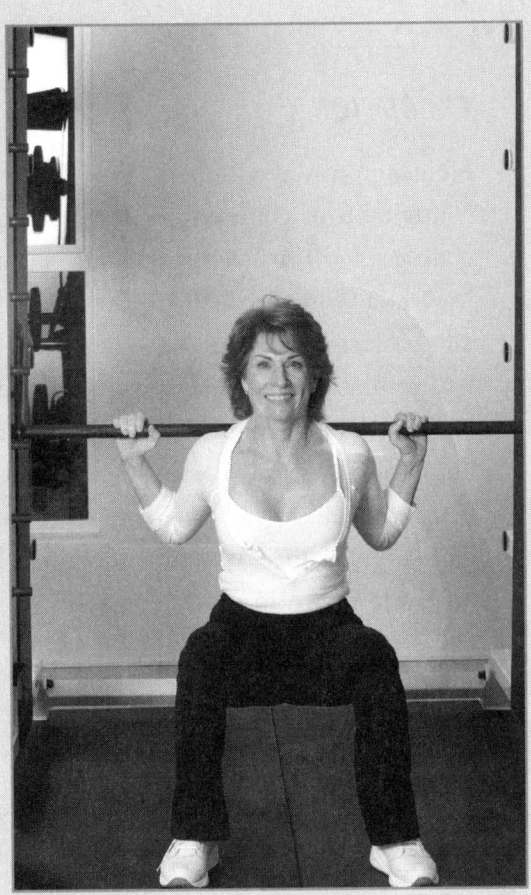

②

Squats on Smith Machine

EXECUTION

A Smith Machine is a machine commonly found in gyms. It has a bar attached to hinges that slide up and down cable wires. Because it is guided movement, it is sometimes a little easier to use than free weight barbells.

Standing in front of the machine, place the bar of the Smith Machine so it rests comfortably on your upper back (trapezius). You should align your legs directly under your hips with your feet facing forward. Your knees should be slightly flexed. Begin with your feet a little wider than hip-distance apart and your abdominal muscles contracted. Lower your body into a squat position, until the front of your legs are at approximately a 90-degree angle at the knee joint. Continue to contract the buttocks (glutes) and the muscles in the front of your leg (quads) as you stand up to starting position from the squat.

Muscles Working:
Buttocks and Front of Legs—
Gluteals and Quadriceps

Degree of Difficulty:
Three Dumbbells

Equipment:
Smith Machine

Body Position:
Standing

Form Watch:
Maintain a tight contraction in your abdominals the entire time and don't allow your knees to go out over your toes.

Standing Side Leg Lifts

Muscles Working:
Sides of the Buttocks
(Gluteus medius)

Degree of Difficulty:
One Dumbbell

Equipment:
None Required

Body Position:
Standing

Form Watch:
Do not allow your
body to tilt to the side,
stand up straight,
shoulders back and
abdominal muscles
contracted.

EXECUTION

You can do this by just placing your hands on your waist, if you have good balance; if not, hold onto a chair, a counter, or any sturdy object for support. Stand tall with your feet placed next to one another, toes parallel. Contract your abdominals tightly. Make sure your hips are aligned, don't allow one to come out in front of the other. Flex the foot of the working leg and bring it away from the stationary leg. Bring the foot as far to the side as your hip range of motion permits. Keep your buttocks contracted and feel a squeeze at the side of your buttocks as well as on the outer thigh muscles. Keeping your foot flexed, slowly return it to the beginning position, leading with the inner thigh. Do not let the foot rest on the floor but immediately bring it back up to the side to complete all repetitions.

Standing Rear Leg Lifts

EXECUTION

Using both hands, hold onto a chair, counter, or tabletop for balance and stability. Tilt your body position so you are at a slight forward angle. Contract your abdominals. With the foot of the working leg flexed, lift the leg straight back behind you, squeezing the buttocks the entire time, then return it to starting position. This is not a wide range of motion exercise. Once started, your foot should not touch the floor until you've completed all your repetitions.

Muscles Working:
Buttocks (Gluteus
Maximus)

Degree of Difficulty:
One Dumbbell

Equipment:
None Required

Body Position:
Standing

Form Watch:
Stand up tall, with
your abdominals
tightly contracted the
entire time and your
shoulders and neck
relaxed.

Stationary Lunges

Muscles Working:
Front of Legs and
Buttocks—
Gluteals and
Quadriceps

Degree of Difficulty:
Three Dumbbells

Equipment:
None Required

Body Position:
Standing

Form Watch:
It is very important
not to let the knee of
your front leg go out
over your toes.

EXECUTION

Stand straight with your abdominals contracted. Your arms are resting comfortably at your sides or around your waist. If you feel uncertain of your balance, you can do lunges holding onto a countertop or sturdy table to keep yourself steady. Bring one leg forward bending your knee and dropping down into a lunge position. The knee of the back leg drops toward the ground into a 90-degree angle. Make sure your front knee does not come out over your toes. Squeeze your buttocks muscles tightly and keep the abdominals contracted the entire time. Hold the lunge position for about 3 to 5 seconds then bring the foot back to starting position. You can do these alternating legs or doing the entire set with the same leg and then switch off and do the next set with the other leg. (See photo on page 68 as an example of proper form and technique for this exercise.)

Reverse Lunges

EXECUTION

Holding onto a stationary object—the bar of a Smith Machine, a door handle, a sturdy table or countertop—stand straight with your abdominals contracted. Bring one leg behind you, bending the knee so your leg is at a 90-degree angle to your body. Your torso should remain tall, back straight, chest open, and head high. From starting position, you lunge backward by bending your front knee into a 90-degree angle without letting your knee come out over your toes. Try and bring your bent back leg so your shin is parallel to the ground. Hold the lunge for about three seconds and return to starting position. (See photo on page 74 as an example of proper form and technique for this exercise.)

Muscles Working:
Buttocks and Front
of Legs—
Gluteals and
Quadriceps

Degree of Difficulty:
Three Dumbbells

Equipment:
None Required

Body Position:
Standing

Form Watch:
Contract your glute
muscles the entire
time and keep your
posture upright.

Sit Downs

Muscles Working:
Buttocks and Front
of Legs—
Gluteals and
Quadriceps

Degree of Difficulty:
One or Two Dumbbells

Equipment:
None

Body Position:
Standing

Form Watch:
Stand tall as you do
the Sit Downs; don't
bow over.

EXECUTION

To do Sit Downs, you can use a hard-surfaced chair in your home or a flat bench in the gym or even a piano bench. The chair should be low enough so you can get a good squat down into it.

Stand in front of the chair or bench a little farther than you would if you were actually going to sit down on it. Place your feet hip-distance apart. You can place your hands in front of your body or folded across your chest.

Bend your knees as if you were going to sit down, but you are only going to touch the surface of the chair with your buttocks and come right back up again.

This is a continuous action exercise so you do not stop between your repetitions.

Treasure Your "Chest"

Builders and Boosters

Life only demands from you the strength you possess . . .
DAG HAMMARSKJOLD

How does your strength fail you? Well, it leaves you unable to perform the activities of daily life that are vital to your well being. Also, it leaves you feeling less of a person. "Am I all the woman I can be?" you might ask yourself. "My energy is flagging. My self esteem is diminishing. I'm losing my sense of spirit and vigor. I'm feeling old. I don't want to lose my sense of spirit. I don't want to feel old."

You probably don't relate these feelings to a loss of muscle and strength, but they are, in both very subtle and dynamic ways.

Anti-Aging Strategy 5 gives you exercises to help preserve your chest muscles, the Pectoralis major and minor. The pec major muscle is your largest chest muscle. You can feel it between your clavicle and your top ribs. The pec major also attaches to your upper arm bone (humerus) and is used powerfully in throwing a ball or playing tennis. The pectoralis minor is a much smaller muscle of the chest wall and does not connect to the arm bone. Both the pec major and minor are also responsible, in part, for holding up our breasts. The stronger these muscles are, the more youthful the body appears and the more beautiful your entire upper body carriage. As we age, we all face that old enemy "gravity" which inevitably tries to "yank" our breasts (not to mention everything else) downward. Muscle is a woman's anti-aging gravity buster!

Body Preserving Exercises—
Chest—Builders and Boosters

1   Chest Flyes Using Dumbbells on Flat Bench
2   Ball Push-Ups
3   Flyes on a Pec Machine
4   Chest Press on Bench Using Body Bar or Smith Machine
5   Dumbbell Presses Over Exercise Ball

Equipment-Free Body Preserving Chest Exercises:

6   Wall Push-Ups
7   Flyes
8   Presses
9   Floor Push-Ups

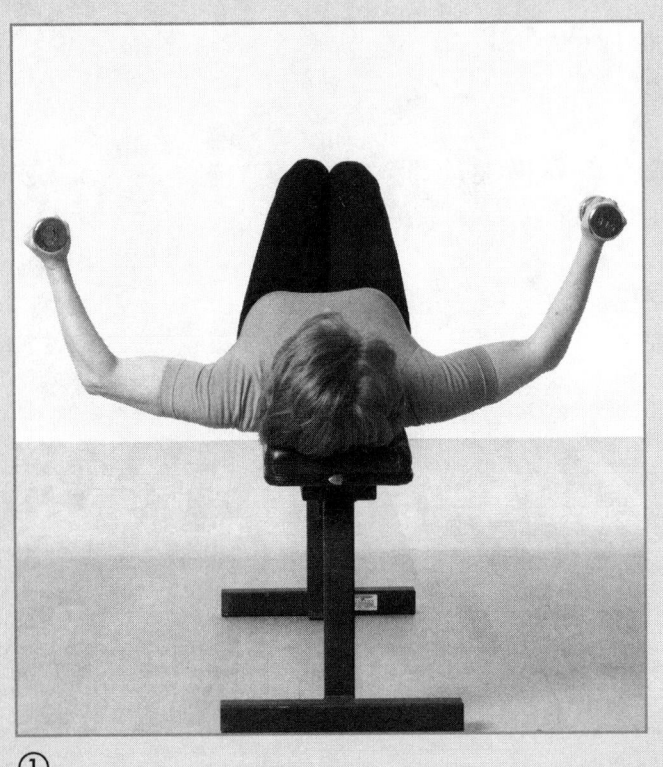

①

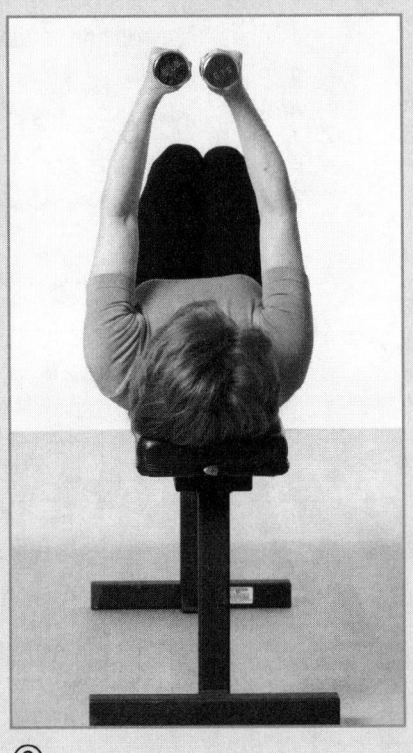

②

Chest Flyes Using Dumbbells on Flat Bench

EXECUTION

Lying on a flat bench, place your feet on the bench away from your body so you're in a comfortable position. Hold the dumbbells so your fingertips are facing inward.

Your arms are open wide so you feel a slight lengthening of the chest muscles even in this starting position.

Slowly bring the dumbbells up toward one another so they will eventually come together above your breast, at the midline of your body.

Bring your arms slowly back to starting position, maintaining the wide arch and feeling the lengthening of your muscles across your chest.

Muscles Working:
Chest (Pectoralis Major and Minor)

Degree of Difficulty:
One Dumbbell

Equipment:
Dumbbells and Flat Bench

Body Position:
Lying on a Flat Bench

Form Watch:
Even though you are lying on a flat bench, keep your abdominals contracted to protect your low back and strengthen your core.

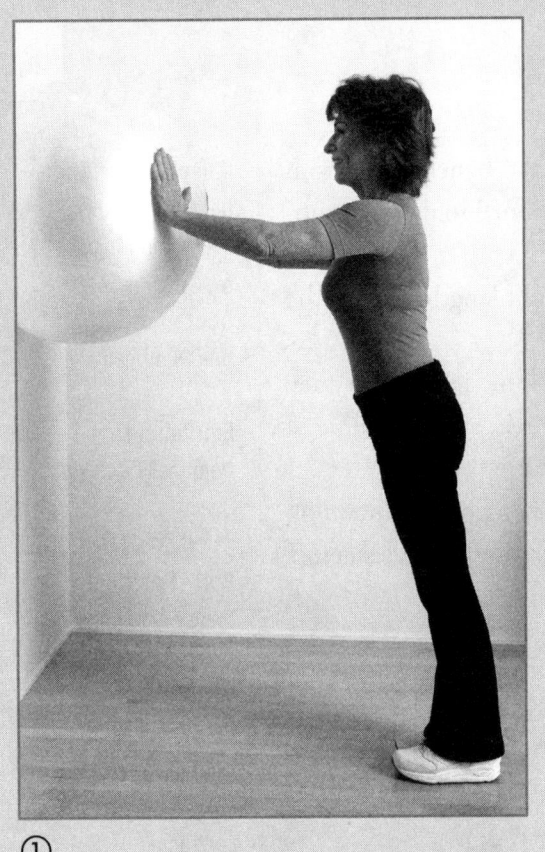

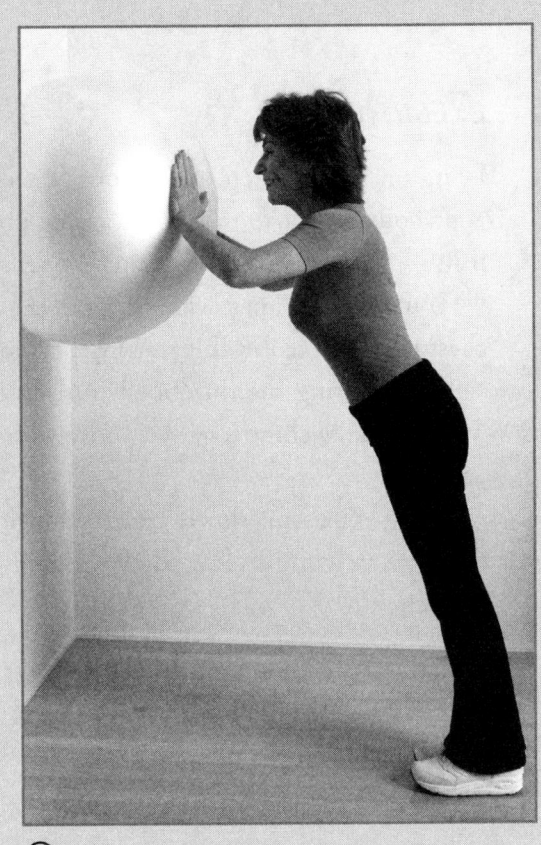

①   ②

Ball Push-Ups

EXECUTION

Place your hands flat against an exercise ball placed against the wall. Your hands are placed about three inches wider than shoulder width. Bring your feet backward so you are leaning slightly toward the ball. Your feet are together placed about twenty-four inches from the wall, so your body is at angle. Your arms are straight with a small bend at the elbow. Your abdominals are tightly contracted.

Bending your elbows deeply, press forward toward the ball, leading with your chest, not your head. Your spine is straight. You will feel a lengthening of your chest muscles as your body leans in.

Without letting your hands shift, push back away from the ball to starting position, maintaining about a 5-degree bend in your elbow.

Muscles Working:
Chest (Pectoralis Major and Minor)

Degree of Difficulty:
One Dumbbell

Equipment:
Exercise Ball

Body Position:
Standing

Form Watch:
Don't drop your head. Your body should remain like a plank, head, neck, and spine in alignment.

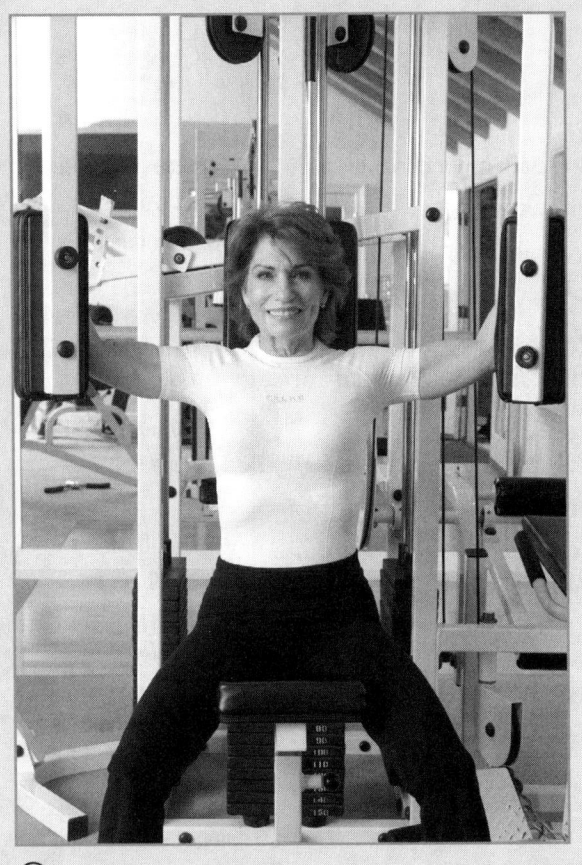

①

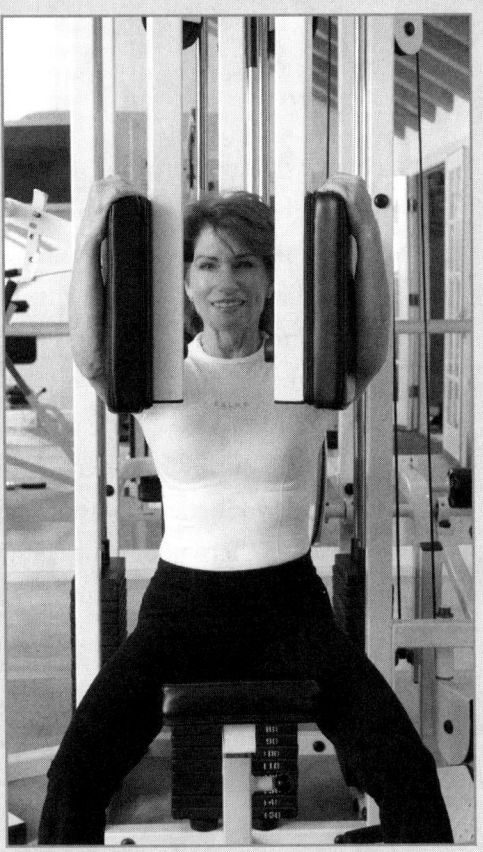

②

Flyes on a Pec Machine

EXECUTION

If the machine has an adjustable seat, raise or lower it so your feet are placed firmly on the floor. Some machines also have adjustable arms. You will want to place your forearms on the pads so your elbows are at a 90-degree angle. In the starting position, your arms should not be so far behind your body that your shoulders are hyperextended, or too far in front that you don't get enough range of motion.

Even though you are in a seated position, contract your abdominals while placing your back flat against the back of the machine. Sit up tall.

Slowly bring your arms together so they meet at your body's midline at the same time. You will feel a contraction in your upper chest.

Release slowly back to starting position. As you do, apply resistance against the arms of the machine. Don't allow the force of the machine to pull you back.

Muscles Working:
Chest (Pectoralis Major and Minor)

Degree of Difficulty:
One Dumbbell

Equipment:
Pec Machine

Body Position:
Seated

Form Watch:
Keep your abdominal muscles contracted the entire time and don't hold any tension in your neck or upper back.

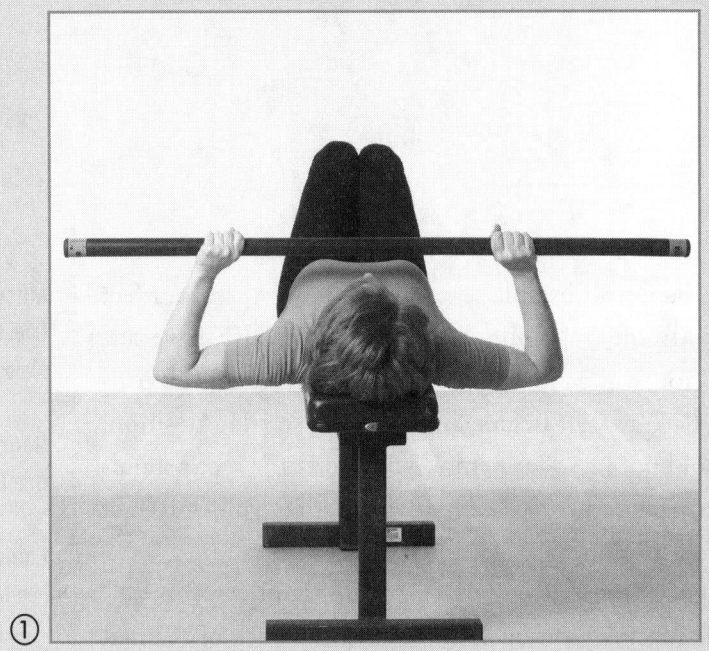

①

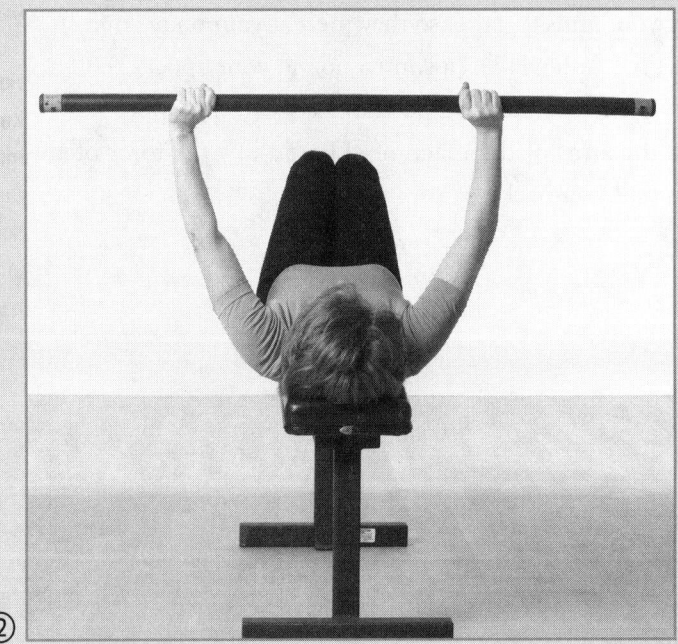

②

Chest Press on Bench Using Body Bar or Smith Machine

EXECUTION

You can do this exercise using a Smith Machine if you are in a gym, or using a body bar (as shown) or barbell either in the gym or at home. The advantage to a Smith Machine is that it is guided movement, so there's no chance of you tipping the bar, as there might be with a barbell. The disadvantage to a Smith Machine is that it is a major piece of equipment so smaller gyms may not have one. The movement you'll be doing—presses—is effectively done either way.

Lying on a flat bench, contract your abdominal muscles. The bar should be placed just above your breast but not at your neck. Hold the body bar, barbell, or the bar of the machine so your hands are wider than shoulder-width apart.

Push the bar up so your arms are almost nearly straight, but maintain a slight bend in your elbow joint. You will feel a contraction across the front of your chest into the front shoulder joint. Slowly lower the bar to starting position without letting it come down too rapidly. Control the movement.

Muscles Working:
Chest (Pectoralis Major and Minor)

Degree of Difficulty:
Two Dumbbells

Equipment:
Barbell or Smith Machine

Body Position:
Lying

Form Watch:
Control the movement of the bar so as you bring it back down toward your chest; you resist against gravity.

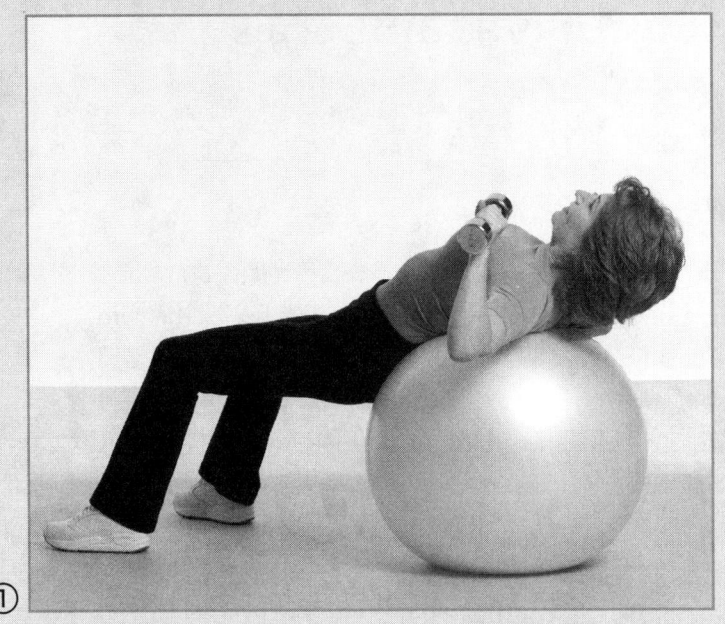

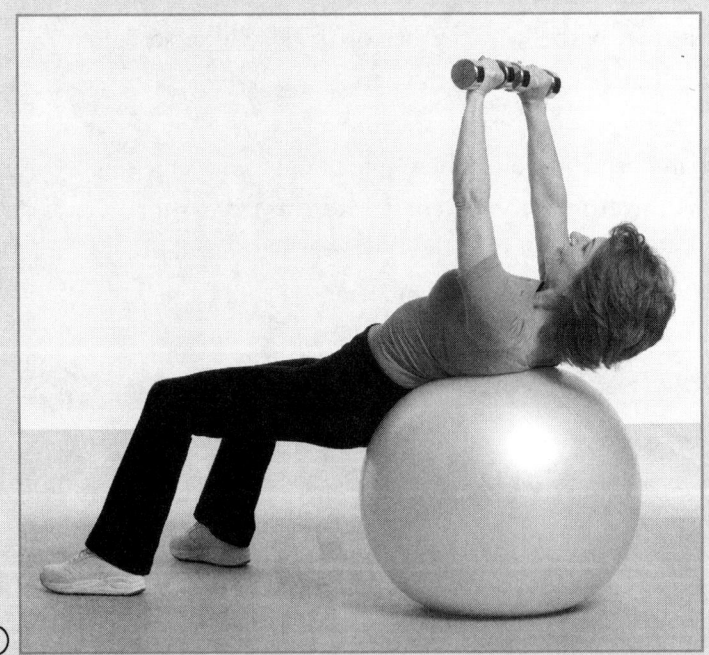

Dumbbell Presses Over Exercise Ball

EXECUTION

Sit on an exercise ball, then lean back slowly arching your body over the ball so your back is resting comfortably on it. Your feet are placed firmly on the ground to prevent the ball from rolling out from underneath you. Contract your abdominal muscles to stabilize your position on the ball. This exercise not only works your chest muscles, but because it is done on a ball, it also helps with your core strengthening.

Hold a pair of dumbbells in your hands so your knuckles are facing up toward the ceiling. Your hands start out parallel to your shoulders, with your elbows pointed toward the ground. Slowly bring the dumbbells up over your body so they meet together right above your chest. You will feel a contraction in your chest muscles. The dumbbells should come together end to end but should not actually touch one another.

Slowly and with control, bring the dumbbells down to starting position parallel with your shoulders. You will feel a lengthening of the muscles across your chest.

Muscles Working:
Chest (Pectoralis Major and Minor)

Degree of Difficulty:
Three Dumbbells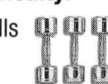

Equipment:
Dumbbells and an Exercise Ball

Body Position:
Lying

Form Watch:
Keep your abdominals tightly contracted the entire time to help insure you remain stable on the ball.

Wall Push-Ups

Equipment-Free Exercises

Muscles Working:
Chest (Pectoralis Major and Minor)

Degree of Difficulty:
One Dumbbell

Equipment:
None Required

Body Position:
Standing

Form Watch:
Keep your abdominal muscles contracted and your body in alignment.

EXECUTION

Stand about twelve to fourteen inches away from a wall. Angle your body toward the wall by placing your hands so they are about an inch wider than and above your shoulder joint. Your fingers should be close together and your fingertips should be facing towards the ceiling. Contract your abdominals before beginning. Slowly and with control, lean your chest toward the wall. Do not lead with your head. Your spine should be straight and your posture upright. As you lean in to the wall your elbows point outward. You will feel a slight contraction across your chest. When you push away from the wall to return to starting position, do not straighten your elbows completely but keep a slight bend in them. (See photo on page 88 as an example of proper form and technique for this exercise.)

Flyes

EXECUTION

You can do these either seated or standing, whatever feels most comfortable for you. Whether you are seated or standing, contract your abdominals. Bring your arms up so your elbows are parallel with your shoulders, forming a 90-degree angle, and your palms are facing forward. Keep your neck relaxed. You will be bringing your arms together, like two swinging doors closing, so they will meet at your body's midline. Lead the movement more with your elbows than the palms of your hands. As you bring the elbows toward one another, you will feel a squeeze in the upper part of your chest. When your elbows touch one another, bring your arms back out again to starting position. (See photo on page 90 as an example of proper form and technique for this exercise.)

Equipment-Free Exercises

Muscles Working:
Chest (Pectoralis Major and Minor)

Degree of Difficulty:
One Dumbbell

Equipment:
None Required

Body Position:
Standing or Seated

Form Watch:
Move slowly and concentrate on feeling the muscles of the chest contracting.

Presses

Muscles Working:
Chest (Pectoralis
Major and Minor)

Degree of Difficulty:
One Dumbbell

Equipment:
None Required

Body Position:
Standing or Seated

Form Watch:
Concentrate on
squeezing the chest
muscles as your arms
move together.

EXECUTION

Presses can be done either seated or standing, whatever feels most comfortable for you. If seated, plant feet firmly on the ground. If standing, place your feet hip-distance apart. Bring your hands up so they are parallel with your shoulders, your fingertips are tucked in forming a lose fist. Shift your elbows so they are not facing toward the floor but pointed at the wall behind, keeping your forearms parallel to the floor. Move your two fists simultaneously toward the midline of your body, leaving enough space between your fists and your body so you could place a beach ball between them. When your fists come together, your thumbs and first fingers should touch, not your knuckles. Be sure to keep your arms at shoulder height. As you return your fists to starting position, lead with your elbows going backward, keeping your chest open and your head straight.

Floor Push-Ups

EXECUTION

Push-ups on the floor can be done with your feet straight out behind you—a full military push up—or with your knees bent
which is called a half push-up. Place your hands about an inch
wider than and just above your shoulders, with your palms flat on
the ground and fingertips pointing sideways. (When your fingertips point sideways in the push-up position, it really focuses the
work on the chest muscles. When your fingertips point forward,
you're working more biceps than chest muscles.) Keep a slight
bend in the elbow. Move toward the ground leading with your
chest. Make certain your spine is straight and that your body is
not sinking in the middle. This is accomplished by keeping abdominals contracted and tight the entire time. Bring your chest
down to the point where there would be enough space to place
your fist between your chest and the ground. That is the ideal
push-up. If you cannot go down that far, go as close to that stan-
dard as possible. Push back up to starting position maintaining a
slight bend at the elbow.

Muscles Working:
Chest (Pectoralis
Major and Minor)

Degree of Difficulty:
Three Dumbbells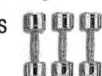

Equipment:
None Required

Body Position:
Prone

Form Watch:
Your head is in
alignment with your
spine so you are not
leading with your chin
or dropping your head
down.

"Back" in Business

Reinforcers and Developers

Once begun a task is easy, half the work is done.

HORACE

Your back muscles comprise some of the largest, and strongest muscles in your upper body. It is critical for women of all ages, but especially those who are starting and going through menopause, to make sure the large muscles of the back stay strong and functional. Unlike men, most women don't always focus on back exercises because we're more concerned with more of the "glamour" areas, like the back of our arms, our waist and stomachs. But believe me, these exercises for your back muscles are essential to keep your body in alignment, protect your posture to help eliminate "stooping," and to increase your entire upper body strength.

The major back muscles are the trapezius muscle, the rhomboid muscles and the latissimus dorsi muscles.

The trapezius muscle, often referred by its nickname "traps," is such a large back muscle, for exercise purposes it is usually divided into the upper fibers, middle fibers, and lower fibers. The main job of your traps is to help elevate and lower your scapulae (shoulder blades) so you can perform such actions as lifting. For instance, your traps would come into play if you were lifting something heavy off the ground with your hands, like a suitcase.

The rhomboid muscles (major and minor) are located in your mid-back on either side of your mid-spine. They are a much smaller muscle than your traps, but they work together to help stabilize your back and assist with upward and downward movements.

Finally, there is the Lastissiumus dorsi, also often referred to by its less formalized name, the lats. They are the only muscle from this group that attaches to the humerus (your arm bone) so it is a big player in arm movement. Whenever you are using your arms to pull something down, a box from the top shelf of your closet, for example, your lats are helping to perform the action.

Especially critical for the menopausal woman is maintaining back and neck range of motion. Equally important is protecting the integrity of the spine by keeping these major muscle groups strong.

The exercises below strengthen and build all your back muscles to keep you structurally strong and functionally fit, so no matter what task of daily living comes your way, you'll be "back in business!"

Body Preserving Exercises:
Back—Reinforcers and Developers

1 Lat Pull-Downs
2 Machine-Assisted Pull-Ups
3 One-Arm Kneeling Rows
4 Bent-Over Body Bar Rows
5 Seated Low Rows

Equipment-Free Body Preserving Back Exercises:

6 Arm Pull-Downs
7 Back Rows

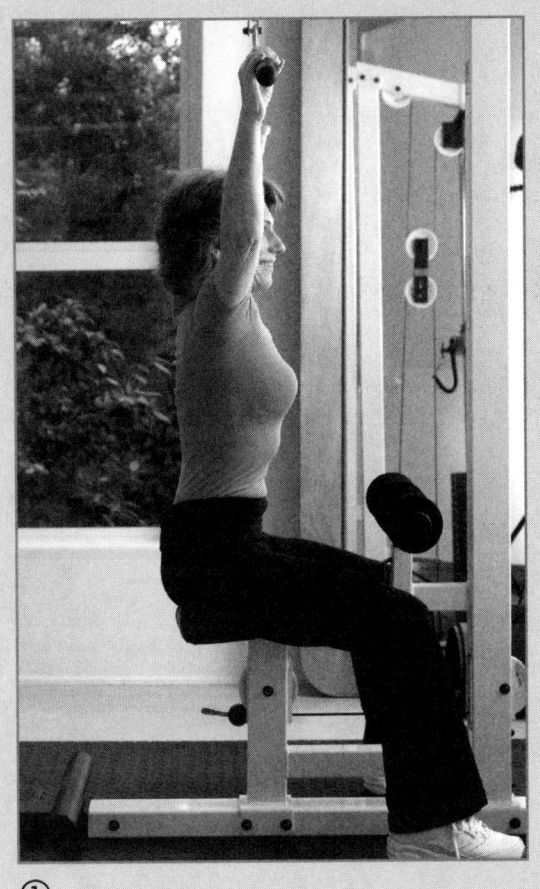

①

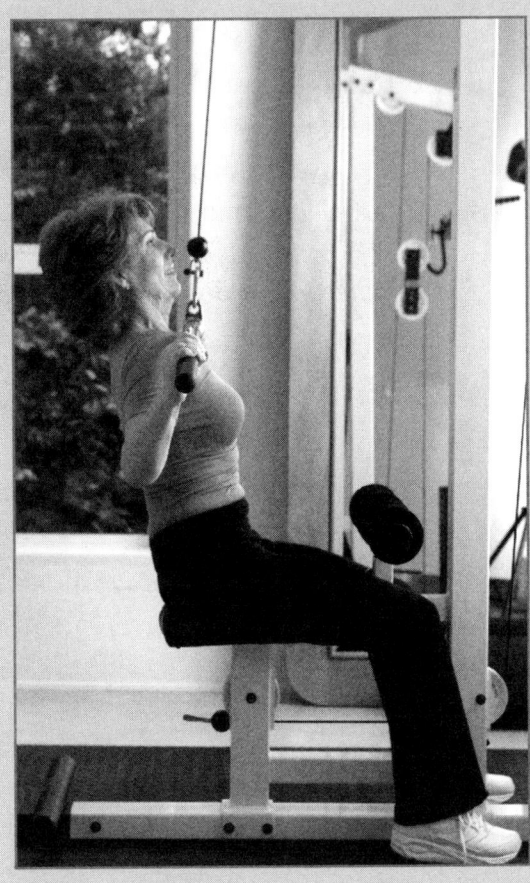

②

Lat Pull-Downs

EXECUTION

The Lat Pull Down Machine is a popular piece of equipment in the gym for working the muscles of the back. It is most frequently a seated piece of equipment with a bar hanging down from a cable above your head.

Sit comfortably on the machine with your knees under the knee hold-down pad. Place your hands on the bar so they are an equal distance apart and the bar is level.

As you pull the bar down toward your upper chest, you lean back slightly while squeezing your back muscles (lats and traps) together. Keep your shoulder blades squeezed together, your spine stabilized, and your abdominals contracted. Continue to contract your lats, and relax your hands and arms as much as possible. Release the bar up slowly to starting position without allowing the gravitational force of the bar to pull you forward.

Muscles Working:
Back—
Traps, Lats,
Rhomboids

Degree of Difficulty:
One Dumbbell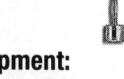

Equipment:
Lat Pull Down
Machine

Body Position:
Sitting on the Machine

Form Watch:
Keep your neck and shoulders relaxed and your abdominals contracted the entire time.

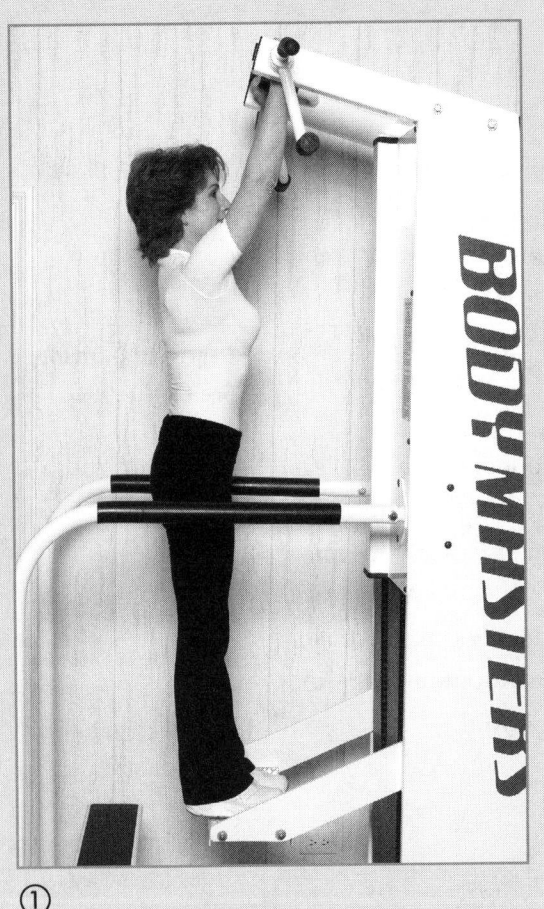

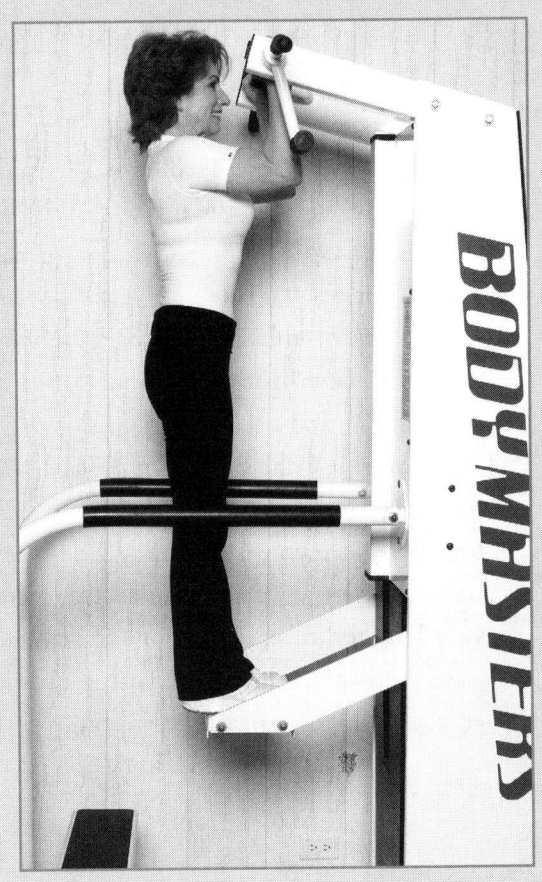

①   ②

Machine-Assisted Pull-Ups

EXECUTION

An assisted pull-up machine allows you to lift your body up into a pull-up that you might not normally be able to do using your own back and arm strength. The machine has handles above your head, a platform and a stack of weights below. You displace your own body weight by selecting an amount of weight you do not want to lift. For example, if you weigh 125 pounds and you select 75 pounds of assistance, you will only be lifting 50 pounds of your own weight.

Stand on the support platform of the machine and grip the bar above your head so you have a firm hold on it. Your arms should be straight but try to keep a slight bend in the elbows. Contract your abdominal muscles and don't let your head drop or have your shoulders pulled up to your ears.

Pull your body upward as high as possible by bending your elbows deeply and contracting your back muscles. Pull your body up until your upper arms are about parallel to the floor. Try to relax your hands and arms as much as possible. As you lower your body to starting position, do not let it fall, but lower with control by continuing to squeeze your back muscles.

Muscles Working:
Back—
Traps, Lats,
Rhomboids

Degree of Difficulty:
Two Dumbbells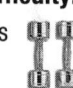

Equipment:
Assisted Pull-Up
Machine (Gravitron)

Body Position:
Standing

Form Watch:
Keep a tight
contraction in your
abdominal muscles
throughout the entire
pull-up action.

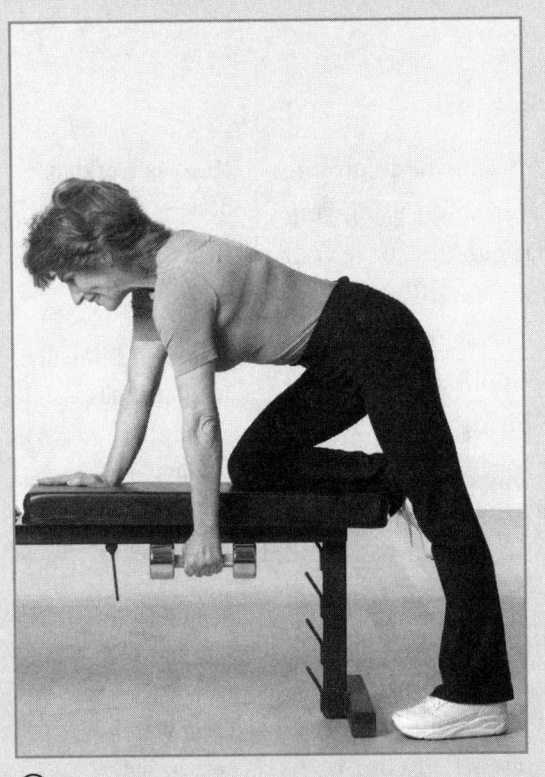

①

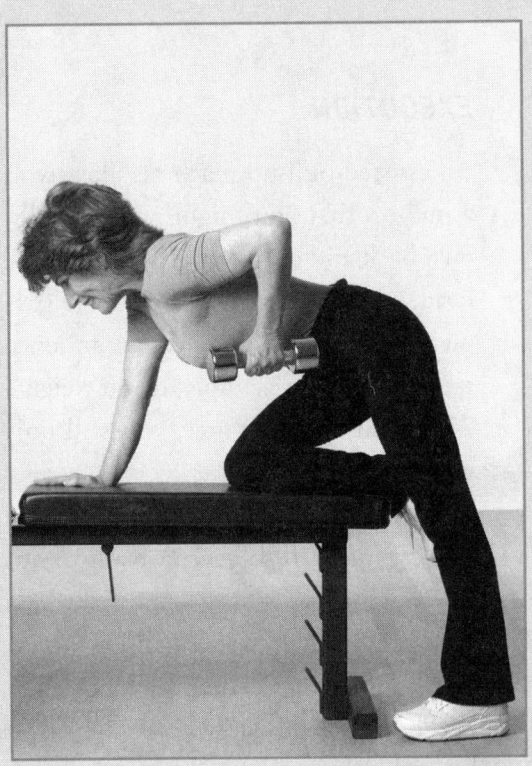

②

One-Arm Kneeling Rows

EXECUTION

You can do these kneeling on a workout bench, but if you're not in a gym or don't own a workout bench, you can do them easily at home by kneeling on chair.

Place one knee on the bench and bend at the waist so your torso is parallel to the floor. Contract your abdominal muscles, which will help protect your core and keep your head in straight alignment with your spine. Do not arch your back or allow your body to droop in the middle.

You will be working the arm by the side of your standing leg. Place the dumbbell in your hand (you can also use a wrist weight) so your fingertips are facing toward the bench and the dumbbell is parallel to your body.

Pull the dumbbell straight up, contracting the back muscles, until your elbow is at a 90-degree angle. You will feel a squeeze in your back muscles.

As you lower the dumbbell to starting position, do not let it simply fall down, but resist against gravity, feeling a lengthening of the back muscles.

Muscles Working:
Back—
Traps, Lats,
Rhomboids

Degree of Difficulty:
Two Dumbbells

Equipment:
Dumbbells

Body Position:
Kneeling on a Flat
Bench

Form Watch:
Don't let the dumbbell
twist in your hand,
control the movement
both going up and
down.

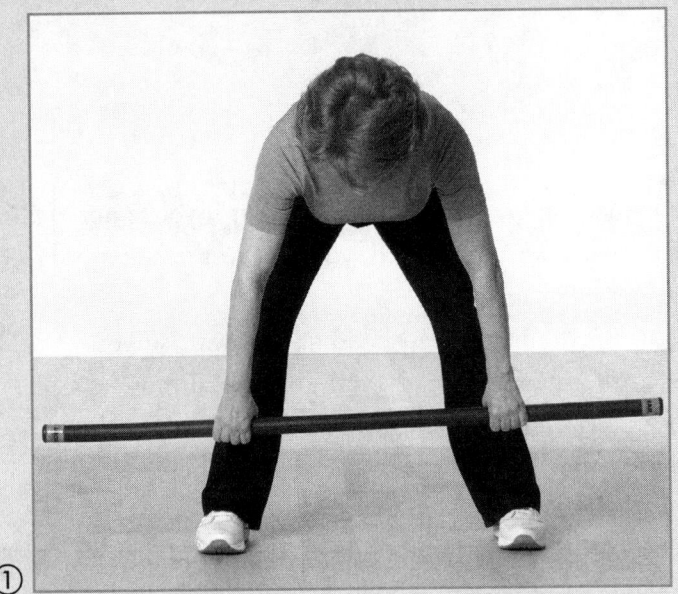

①

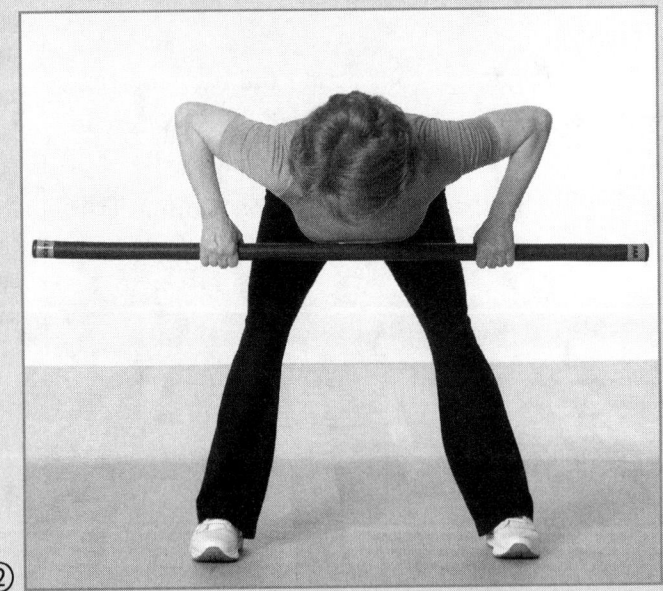

②

Bent-Over Body Bar Rows

EXECUTION

Holding the body bar between your hands evenly balanced, place your feet a little wider than shoulder-width apart and contract your abdominals.

Flex forward at your waist so your torso is parallel to the ground. The bar is hanging in front of you. In this position, your knees should be slightly bent and your abdominals remain very tightly contracted. Do not arch your back. Your head should be in alignment with your spine.

From this position, contract your back muscles together and slowly raise the bar toward your chest by bending your elbows deeply until they reach a 90-degree angle.

As you lower the bar back to starting position, do so slowly by controlling the movement and feel the muscles of the back lengthening.

Muscles Working:
Back—
Traps, Lats,
Rhomboids

Degree of Difficulty:
Three Dumbbells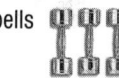

Equipment:
Body Bar or Barbell

Body Position:
Standing

Form Watch:
While in the bent-over position, keep your spine straight and your knees slightly flexed.

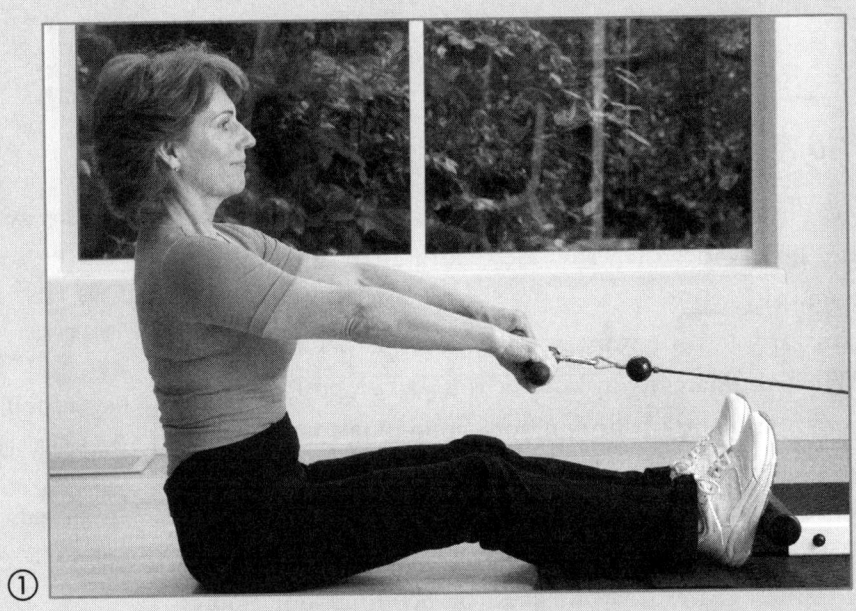

①

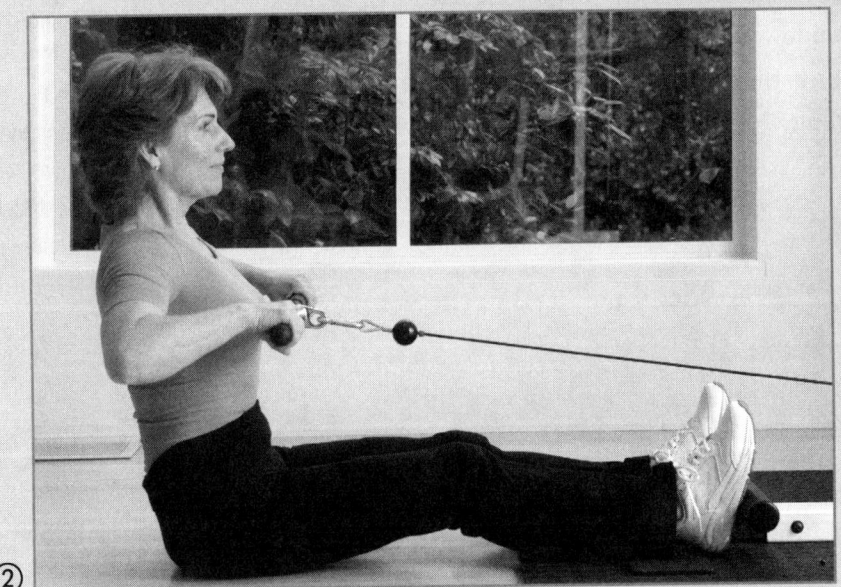

②

Seated Low Rows

EXECUTION

Seated in front of the machine so your arms are outstretched in front of your body, hold the bar between your hands, contract your abdominal muscles, and sit up straight. Your legs are straight out in front of you, but maintain a slight 5-degree bend in your knees so they are not locked out.

Contract your back muscles by squeezing your shoulder blades together and pull the bar toward your body so it is angled toward the middle of your chest. Your elbows bend deeply and are pointed behind your back.

As you release the bar to starting position, do not let it pull your body forward but control the move by maintaining the contraction in your back muscles. Also, as you release to starting position, do not let your body slump forward; maintain an upright posture.

Muscles Working:
Back—
Traps, Lats, Rhomboids

Degree of Difficulty:
Two Dumbbells

Equipment:
Low Row Cable Machine

Body Position:
Seated

Form Watch:
Posture is very important while doing this exercise. It will be easier to maintain the proper body position if you concentrate on keeping your abdominals contracted the entire time.

Arm Pull-Downs

Muscles Working:
Back—
Trapezius,
Rhomboids, Lats

Degree of Difficulty:
One Dumbbell

Equipment:
None Required

Body Position:
Seated or Standing

Form Watch:
Lean slightly forward
and resist against
gravity by keeping
your muscles
isometrically
contracted.

EXECUTION

Arm Pull Downs can be done either seated or standing. If standing, place your feet shoulder-width apart. If seated, sit up straight without resting your back on the chair, giving yourself enough room to move your arms slightly behind your body. Keep abdominals contracted throughout the exercise. To start this exercise, bring your arms in a wide arc above your head. Your hands are forming fists and are coming together so your thumbs are side by side. Keeping your arms away from your body, bring them down leading with your elbows and angling the elbows towards your back. You should feel a squeeze between your shoulder blades as you do this. Return to starting position by slowly controlling the upward move as you go by keeping the muscles contracted.

Back Rows

EXECUTION

You can do Back Rows either seated or standing. If standing, place your feet shoulder-width apart. If seated, sit up straight without resting your back on the chair and giving yourself enough room to move your arms behind you. Keep abdominals contracted throughout the exercise. Bring your arms up alongside your body so your elbows are at a 90-degree angle. Your hands are in line with the middle part of your chest, forming fists with the fingertips facing toward the floor. From starting position, bring your elbows back behind you as if you were rowing a boat, squeezing your shoulder blades together. Do not elevate your shoulders and keep your neck relaxed.

Muscles Working:
Back—
Trapezius,
Rhomboids, Lats

Degree of Difficulty:
One Dumbbell

Equipment:
None Required

Body Position:
Seated or Standing

Form Watch:
Concentrate on contracting the back muscles without any tension in your neck and shoulders.

Up in "Arms"
Definers and Refiners

The secret of success is constancy to purpose.
BENJAMIN DISRAELI

For women, as we become older, our arms become one of those areas we are most embarrassed about . . . especially the back of the arms (triceps). Weak triceps often get called various unflattering names such as "wings," "granny arms," or "that disgusting, flabby under-arm stuff." When I do a class or lecture, one of the most sought after exercises women ask me about are ones that will help them target what I call "the triceps tragedy." The triceps is a three-headed muscle whose job it is to *extend* your elbow; for instance, you'd be using your triceps if you were scratching your back with a back scratcher.

The front of your arm contains the biceps muscles. These are the muscles that *flex* your elbow joint. One of the reasons your biceps muscles might not lose their tone as quickly throughout the aging process as the triceps is that they are used frequently to perform activities of daily life, such as lifting up children, bottles of water, and groceries or lifting your hand to put on lipstick. (I'm not suggesting putting on lipstick is an exercise that will build muscle; it just involves flexing your elbow to get the lipstick to the lips.)

By performing these exercises, described in Anti-Aging Strategy 7, not only will your arms look more beautiful and youthful, you will be building and retaining vital arm strength.

Body Preserving Exercises—
Up in Arms—Defines and Refiners

1 Biceps Curls Using Dumbbells
2 Seated One-Arm Biceps Curls
3 Body Bar Biceps Curls
4 Cable Biceps Curls
5 Triceps Extension Pull Downs
6 Lying Triceps Extension (French Curl)
7 One-Arm Overhead Triceps Extension (French Curl)

Equipment-Free Body Preserving Arm Exercises:

8 Isometric Biceps Curls
9 Triceps Wall Push-Ups
10 Overhead Triceps Extensions
11 Triceps V-Backs

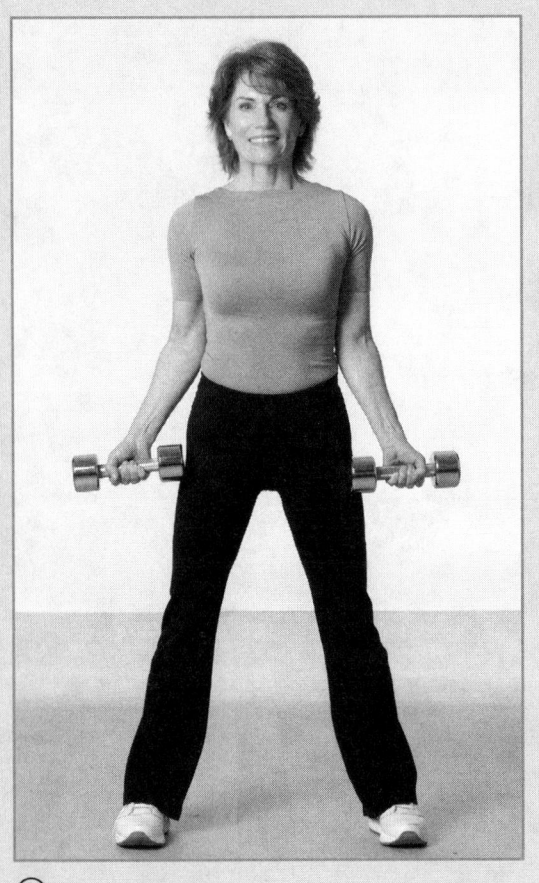

①

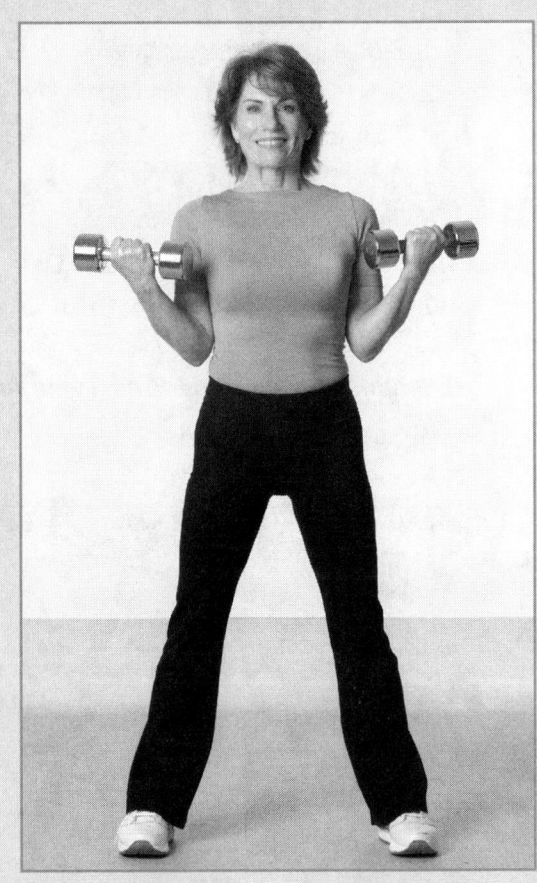

②

Biceps Curls Using Dumbbells

EXECUTION

You need a good, strong base to do biceps curls correctly. Plant your feet firmly on the ground, shoulder-width apart, and contract your abdominal muscles. Keep your knees just slightly bent. Hold a dumbbell in each hand with your fingertips facing away from your body. The sides of the dumbbells start parallel to the top of your thighs (depending on your arm length). To a count of six, slowly perform the "curl" (the action of bringing the dumbbells up to the tops of your shoulders) without moving the arm from its position by the sides of your ribs. Contract the biceps muscles as your bring the dumbbells up.

Release the dumbbells back to starting position, also slowly to a count of six, so you feel a lengthening action of the biceps muscles working against the pull of gravity.

Muscles Working:
Front of Arms—
Biceps

Degree of Difficulty:
One Dumbbell

Equipment:
Dumbbells

Body Position:
Standing

Form Watch:
Do not allow your arms to move from your sides and don't let the dumbbells twist in your hands. Hold them steady.

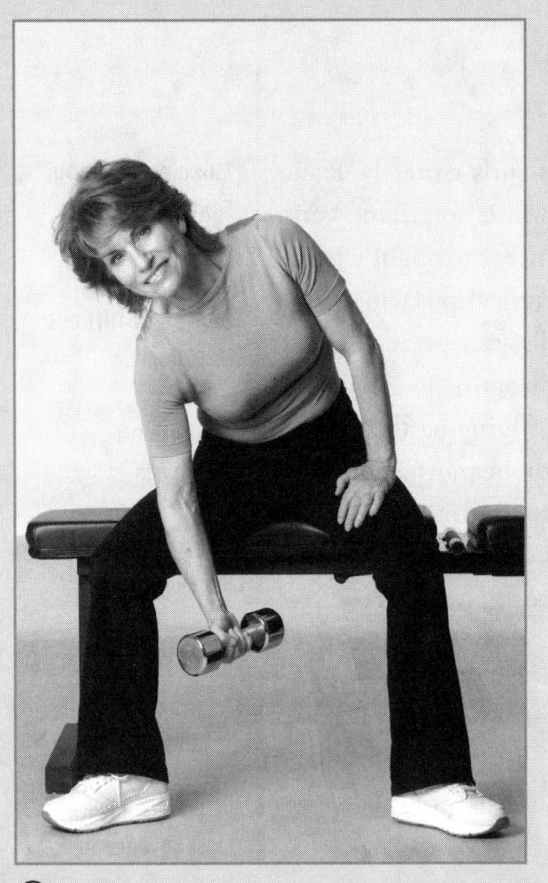

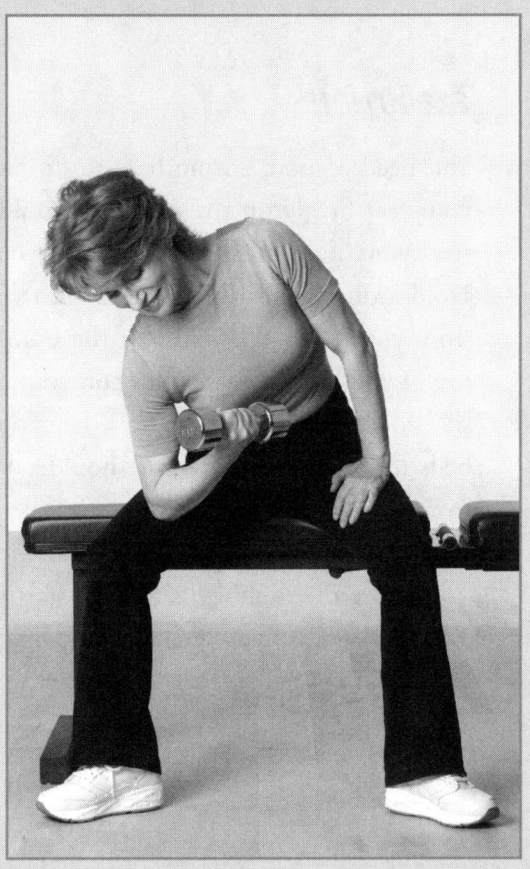

① ②

Seated One-Arm Biceps Curls

EXECUTION

Doing biceps curls one arm at a time allows you to really focus your effort on the individual biceps you are working. If you have one arm that is inherently weaker than the other, working them one at a time will help you strengthen the weaker biceps.

If you are doing these at home, sit on a hard-surface chair. At the gym, sit on a workout bench. Place your feet wide enough apart to allow your torso to lean forward and rest the elbow of the working arm on your inner thigh, just above the knee.

Holding the dumbbell firmly in your hand so it does not twist or turn, you start with your elbow fully extended so your arm is hanging straight down between your legs.

Slowly, to a count of six, curl the dumbbell upward toward your shoulder using a full range of motion, contracting the biceps muscle the entire time. Do not rest at the top of the movement but slowly release the dumbbell back to starting position also to a count of six.

Muscles Working:
Front of Arms—
Biceps

Degree of Difficulty:
Two Dumbbells

Equipment:
Dumbbells

Body Position:
Seated

Form Watch:
As you release the dumbbell, keep the biceps fully contracted, resisting against the pull of gravity, feeling the lengthening of the muscle.

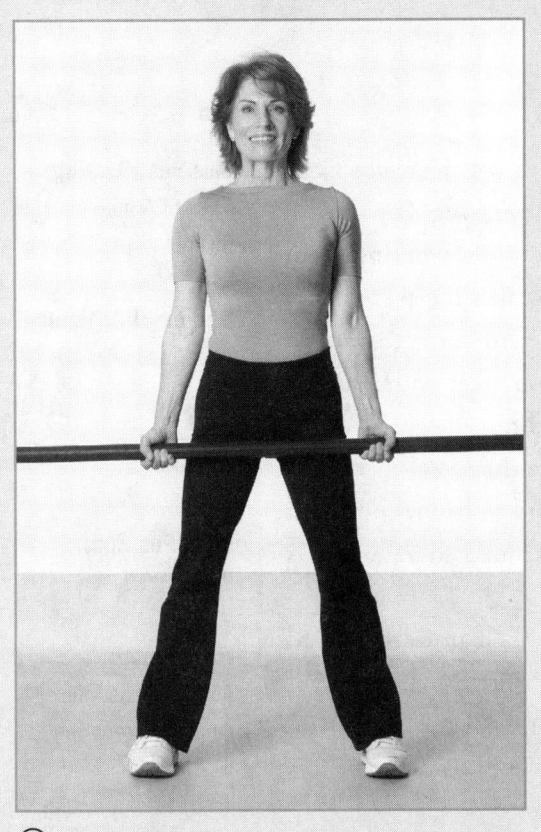

①

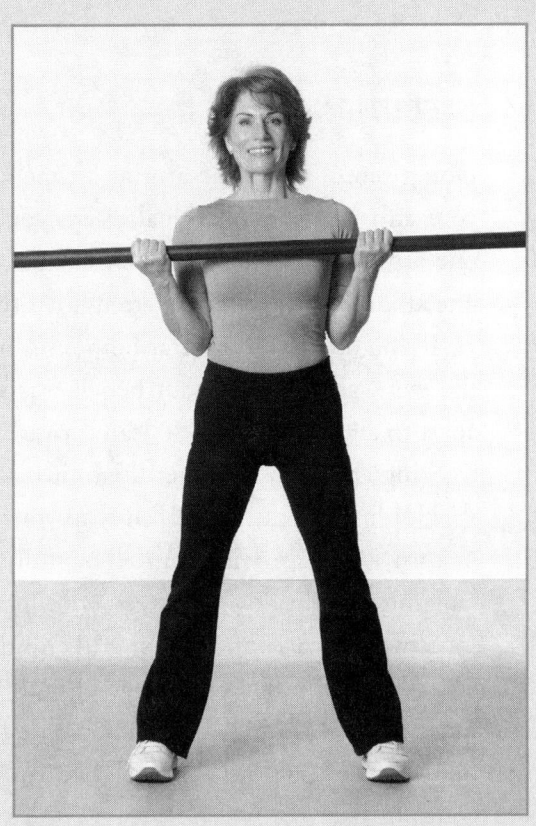

②

Body Bar Biceps Curls

EXECUTION

Hold a body bar or barbell evenly balanced between your two hands so it is at a level angle and your hands are a little wider than shoulder-width apart. Your fingertips are facing outward so your wrists are in neutral position. Posture and stance are very important when you're doing bar biceps curls so plant your feet firmly on the ground, a little wider than hip-distance apart with your abdominal muscles contracted. Your knees should have a slight bend in them, about 5-degrees. Also, to stabilize your core, contract your buttocks.

Holding the bar in front of you, contract your biceps muscles and slowly curl the bar up toward your shoulders, keeping it level the entire time. Release slowly to starting position maintaining the contraction in your biceps and resisting against the natural pull of gravity so you feel the lengthening action of your muscles.

Muscles Working:
Front of Arms—
Biceps

Degree of Difficulty:
Two Dumbbells

Equipment:
Body Bar

Body Position:
Standing

Form Watch:
Hold the bar tightly but do not squeeze it so tightly you are using all your energy to grip the bar rather than perform the exercise.

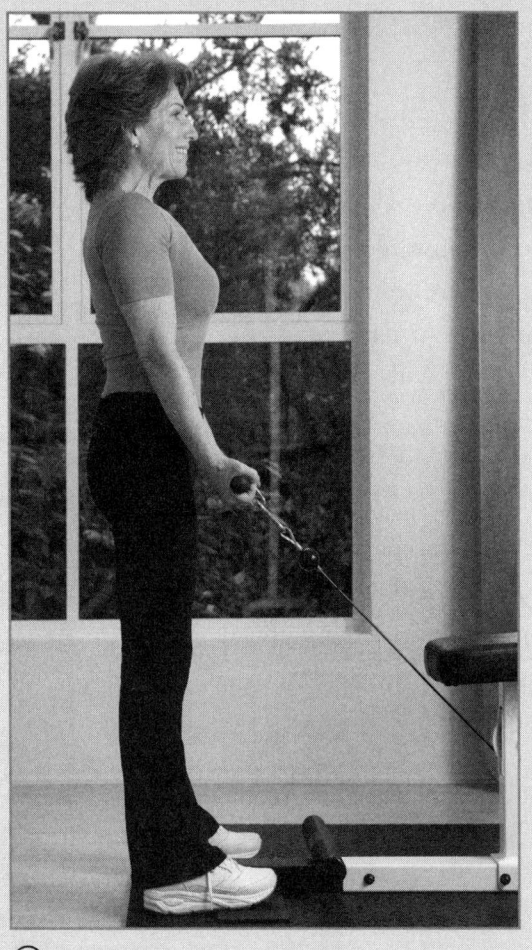

①

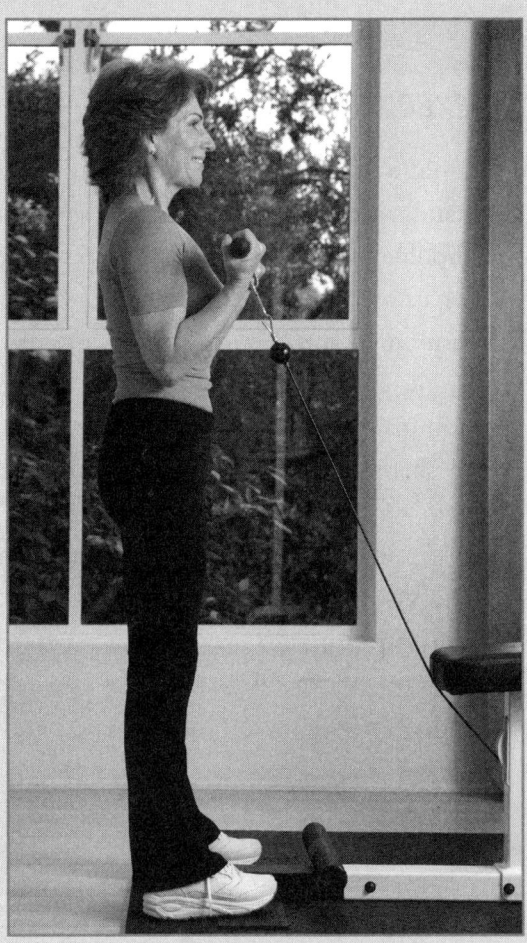

②

Cable Biceps Curls

EXECUTION

This is a standing exercise that requires a good, solid base, so stand with your feet about shoulder-width apart and your knees and hips slightly bent. Your abdominals remain contracted the entire time. Hold the bar attached to the cable evenly balanced between your hands with the inside of your upper arms pulled close in by the sides of your body.

Curl up the bar up by flexing your elbows and contracting your biceps. Do not allow your upper arms to swing with the movement; they remain close to the inside of your upper body. Slowly lower the bar with control to starting position, resisting against the gravitational pull.

Muscles Working:
Front of Arms—
Biceps

Degree of Difficulty:
Three Dumbbells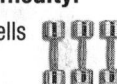

Equipment:
Cable Machine

Body Position:
Standing

Form Watch:
As you curl and release the bar, keep it level so you are not leading with one hand or the other. Don't let the force of the bar pull you out of proper body alignment.

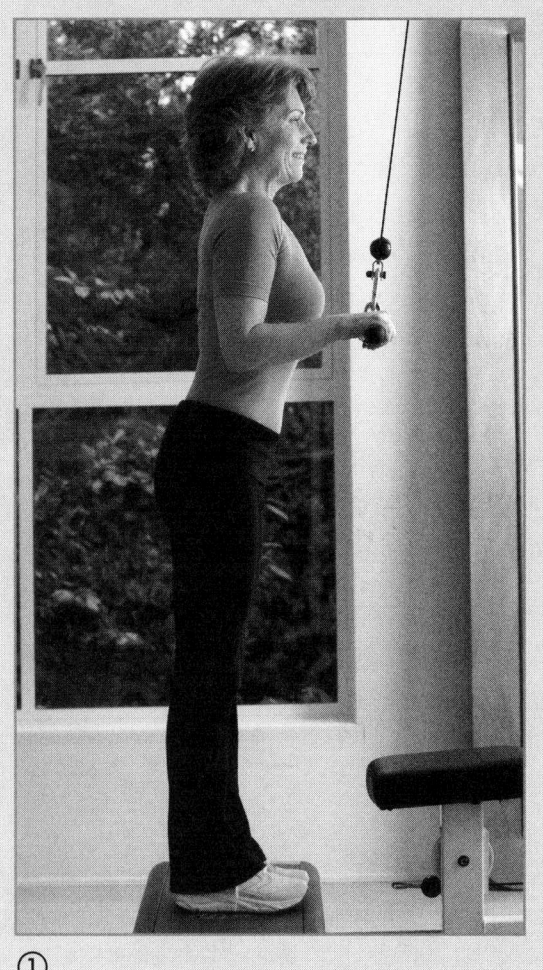

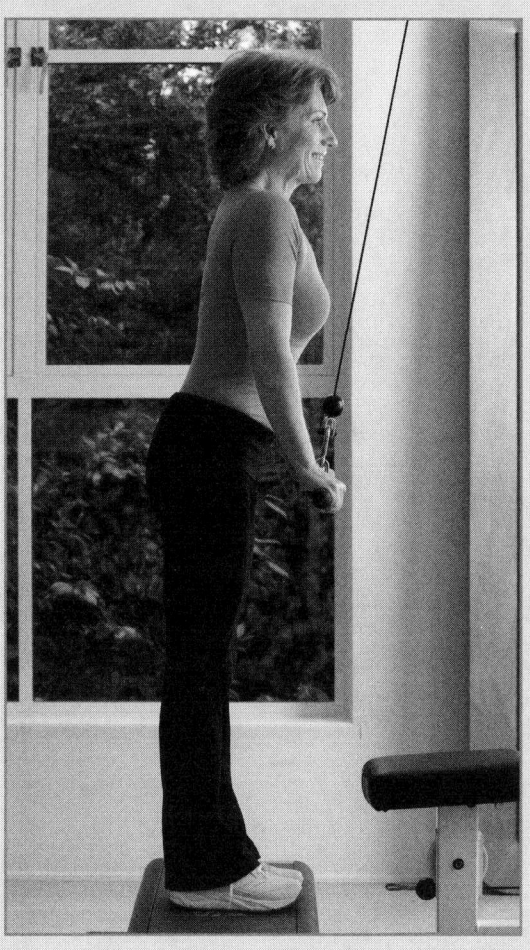

①   ②

Triceps Extension Pull Downs

EXECUTION

The machine on which to do your Triceps Extension Pull Downs has a cable and a short bar hanging from it that will be above your head.

Facing the machine, stand with your feet a little wider than shoulder-width apart and your abdominals tightly contracted to create a firm base. Pull down the bar and hold it in front of you about mid-chest and so it is evenly balanced between your two hands. In starting position your elbows will be bent in a 90-degree angle. From this position, slowly pull the bar down so your arms are straight, maintaining a slight bend at the elbow joint. As you release the bar up to starting position, resist against the natural force of gravity, feeling the lengthening of the triceps muscles in the back of your arms. Keep the insides of your arms glued to your ribs and do not let the bar come up above your mid-chest.

Muscles Working:
Back of Arms—
Triceps

Degree of Difficulty:
One Dumbbell

Equipment:
Cable Machine

Body Position:
Standing

Form Watch:
As you pull down the bar, make sure to keep a very tight contraction in the back of your arms and don't rush the upward movement.

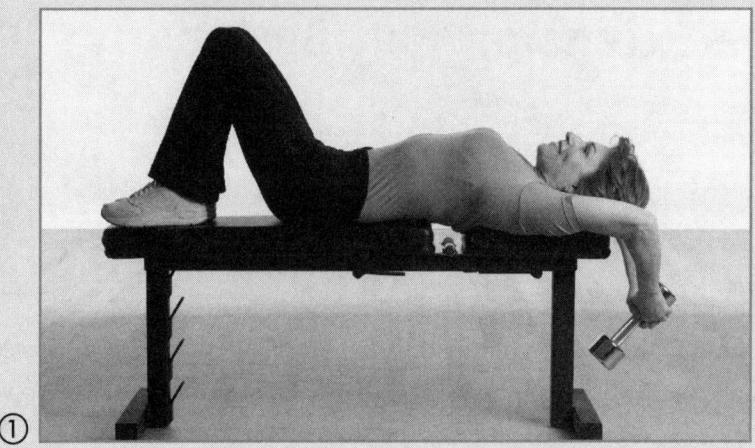

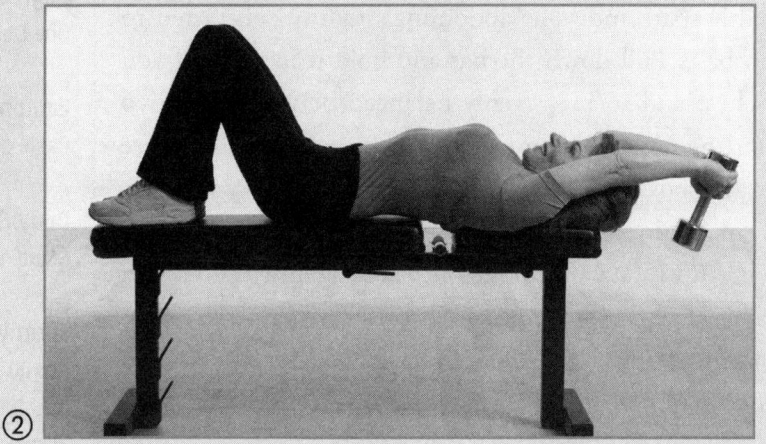

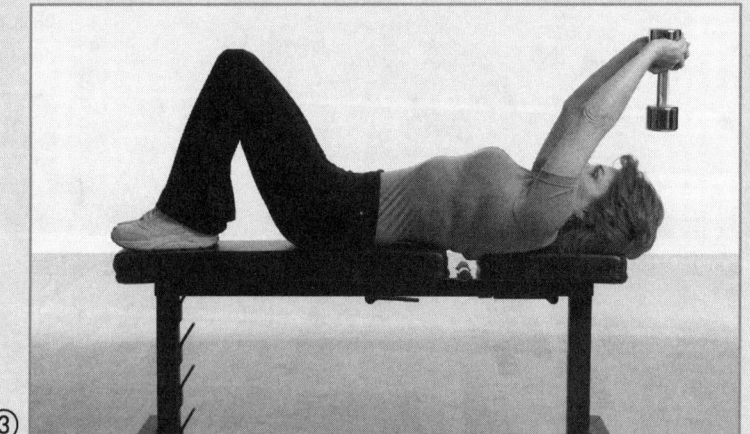

One-Arm Overhead Triceps Extension (French Curl)

EXECUTION

Whether you are standing or sitting, body alignment is very important. If you are standing, create a solid base by keeping your abdominals tightly contracted, feet firmly planted on the ground and hip-distance apart with your knees slightly bent. If you are seated, sit up tall, spine straight, abdominals contracted.

Holding a dumbbell securely in one hand, by its top, not the shaft, carefully place your arm by the side of your head next to your ear. Your elbow should have a deep bend so the dumbbell almost reaches to the top of your back. In this position, you will feel a strong stretch in the back of your arm. Slowly bring the dumbbell straight up behind you and away from your head, squeezing the muscle so you feel a contraction in the back of your arm.

On the release back to starting position, do not let the dumbbell drop with the force of gravity, but resist against it, controlling the movement by keeping the triceps contracted.

Muscles Working:
Back of Arms—
Triceps

Degree of Difficulty:
Three Dumbbells

Equipment:
Dumbbell

Body Position:
Standing or Sitting

Form Watch:
Keep your neck and shoulders relaxed and your spine straight.

Isometric Biceps Curls

Muscles Working:
Front of Arms—
Biceps

Degree of Difficulty:
One Dumbbell

Equipment:
None Required

Body Position:
Seated or Standing

Form Watch:
You must squeeze the muscles the entire time so that it feels the same as if you had a weight in your hand, but you don't.

EXECUTION

Biceps curls can be done seated or standing. If standing, place your feet shoulder-width apart. If seated, sit up straight, feet firmly planted on the ground. Abdominals are contracted and spine is straight. Place your hands by your sides, down by your thighs, rotating your wrists so your fingertips are facing forward. Keep neck and shoulders relaxed. Squeeze your hands into tight fists and keep that contraction which you will feel up the front of your arm. To a count of six, slowly flex your elbow by bringing your closed fists towards your shoulders without taking your arms away from the sides of your body. Throughout the entire movement you isometrically squeeze the muscles so they stay in a constant contraction. Holding that muscle tension constantly, lower your fists to starting position at the sides of your thighs.

Triceps Wall Push-Ups

EXECUTION

Stand about twelve to fourteen inches away from a wall. Place your hands together on the wall so your thumbs are touching and the rest of your fingers are spread out wide, with all fingertips but the thumb pointing toward the ceiling. The inner part of your arms is tight into your body. Your hands should be placed on the wall so they are directly in front of your shoulders. Contract your abdominals before beginning. Move your chest toward the wall keeping your arms locked tightly into the sides of your body. You will feel a strong contraction behind your arms. When you push away from the wall to return to starting position, do not straighten your elbows completely but keep a slight bend in them. (See photo on page 88 as an example of the proper body position to do this exercise.)

Muscles Working:
Back of Arms—
Triceps

Degree of Difficulty:
Two Dumbbells

Equipment:
None Required

Body Position:
Standing

Form Watch:
Do not lead with your head; keep it in alignment with your spine.

Overhead Triceps Extension

Muscles Working:
Back of Arms—
Triceps

Degree of Difficulty:
One Dumbbell

Equipment:
None Required

Body Position:
Seated or Standing

Form Watch:
Don't let your arm
shift from side to side
as you raise it above
your head. Keep it
strong and steady.

EXECUTION

These can be done either seated or standing. If seated, plant feet firmly on the ground. If standing, place your feet hip-distance apart. Keep abdominals contracted to protect your lower back whether you are seated or standing. Raise your arm up and hold your elbow close to your head by the side or behind your ear, until you feel a nice stretch behind the back of your arm. Your hand is almost touching the top of the back of your shoulder. Extend your elbow so your arm comes straight up and slightly behind your head. You must squeeze your muscles the entire time to feel the contraction behind your arm. As you slowly lower your arm back to starting position, feel the lengthening stretch of your muscles as your hand is coming back down to just above your shoulder by the side of your head. Keep it strong and steady. (See photo on page 132 as an example of proper form and technique for this exercise.)

Triceps V-Backs

EXECUTION

Stand with your feet shoulder-width apart, abdominals contracted, spine straight. Start with your hands at mid chest. Your hands should be touching knuckles to knuckles or fists facing one another. The insides of your arms should be hugging your body, firmly pressing against your rib cage. Keep your shoulders relaxed. From the starting position, both fists touching at mid-chest, slowly straighten your elbows bringing your arms back behind you, making the shape of a "V" with your fists as you go back. Keep your triceps muscles contracted as you slowly move your arms behind your body. Slowly return to starting position, fists touching mid-body at your rib cage.

Equipment-Free Exercises

Muscles Working:
Back of Arms—
Triceps

Degree of Difficulty:
One Dumbbell

Equipment:
None Required

Body Position:
Standing

Form Watch:
Maintain good form by keeping your arms at the sides of your body and squeezing the triceps muscles when your arm is straight behind your body.

Straight from the "Shoulders"

Enhancers and Strengtheners

8

I ask not for a lighter burden, but for broader shoulders . . .

JEWISH PROVERB

Vogue Magazine once proclaimed a woman's shoulders one of the sexiest parts of her body. A woman in possession of beautiful shoulders certainly commands attention. The celebrated American society portrait painter, John Singer Sargent, often painted women with their shoulders exposed. Shoulders not only are a striking part of a women's body, but they also provide structural strength to our entire upper body and direct how we carry ourselves.

The main muscle of your shoulder joint is called the deltoid muscle. The front (anterior) fibers of the deltoid muscle allow you to flex and rotate your arm internally and bring it across your body horizontally, for instance, if you were reaching across your body to adjust your bra strap. The back (posterior) fibers extend and externally rotate your arm and allow you to move it horizontally out to the side, like the arm signal you use when driving indicating you'll be turning left.

[139]

To strengthen the entire deltoid muscle, we work the lateral (top) part, the front, and the back. The Body Preserving Exercises that follow target all three areas of your deltoid muscle.

Body Preserving Exercises— Straight from the Shoulders: Enhancers and Strengtheners

1 Side Arm Raises Using Dumbbells

2 One-Arm Front Delt Lifts Using Dumbbells

3 Overhead Presses Using Dumbbells

4 Angled One-Arm Side Raises

5 Shoulder Press Machine

6 Reverse Flyes on Ball Using Dumbbells

Equipment-Free Body Preserving Shoulder Exercises:

7 Side Lateral Arm Raises

8 Overhead Shoulder Presses

9 Reverse Flyes

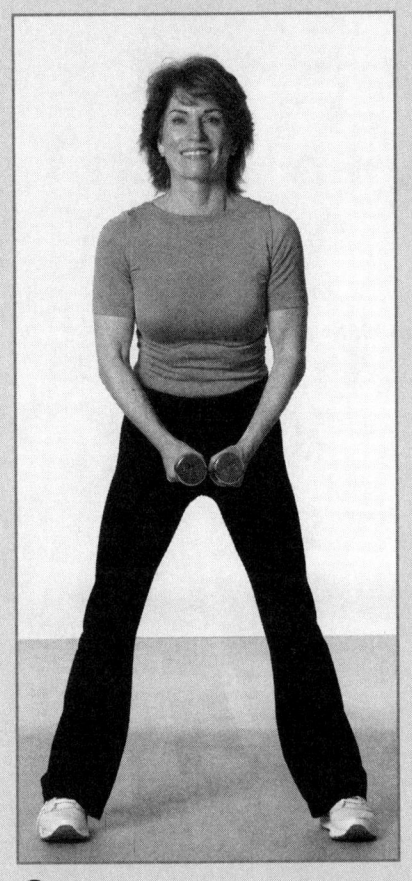
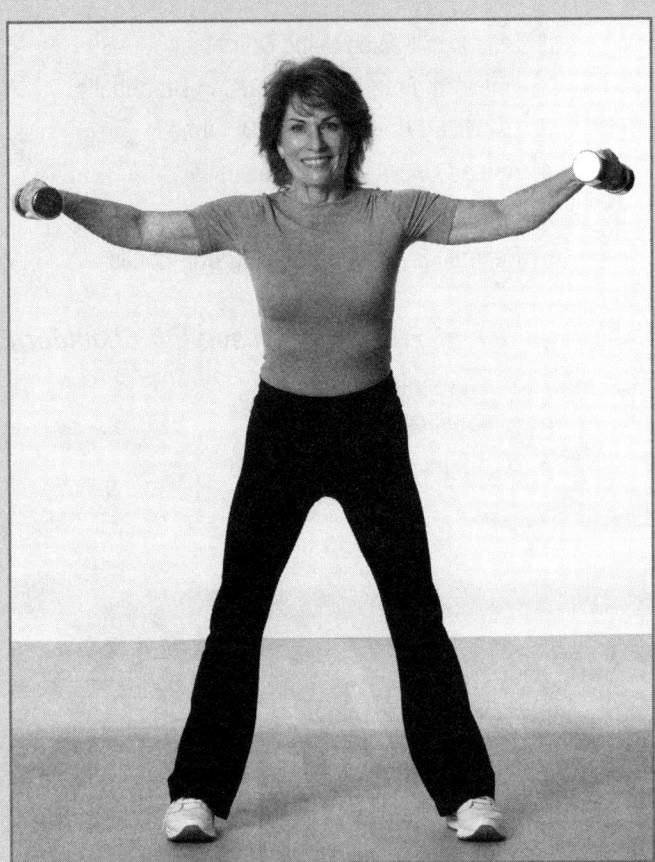

① ②

Side Arm Raises Using Dumbbells

EXECUTION

You can do these Side Arm Raises either standing or sitting. If you are standing, plant your feet firmly on the ground, feet a little wider than hip-distance apart, abdominal muscles tightly contracted. Hold the dumbbells firmly in your hands, fingertips facing toward your body and hanging in front of your pelvic bone. If you are seated, sit up tall, spine straight, abdominals contracted, in a chair without arms or on an exercise bench, so your arms can move freely. The dumbbells are parallel to your thighs and your fingertips are facing toward your body.

Slowly raise the dumbbells out to the sides, like a bird spreading its wings. Stop when they are just parallel to the tops of your shoulders. As you release the dumbbells down to starting position, do so slowly, resisting against gravity and feel a strong lengthening at the top of the shoulders.

Muscles Working:
Shoulders (Lateral Deltoid)

Degree of Difficulty:
One Dumbbell

Equipment:
Dumbbells

Body Position:
Standing or Sitting

Form Watch:
Keep your neck relaxed and your abdominal muscles contracted.

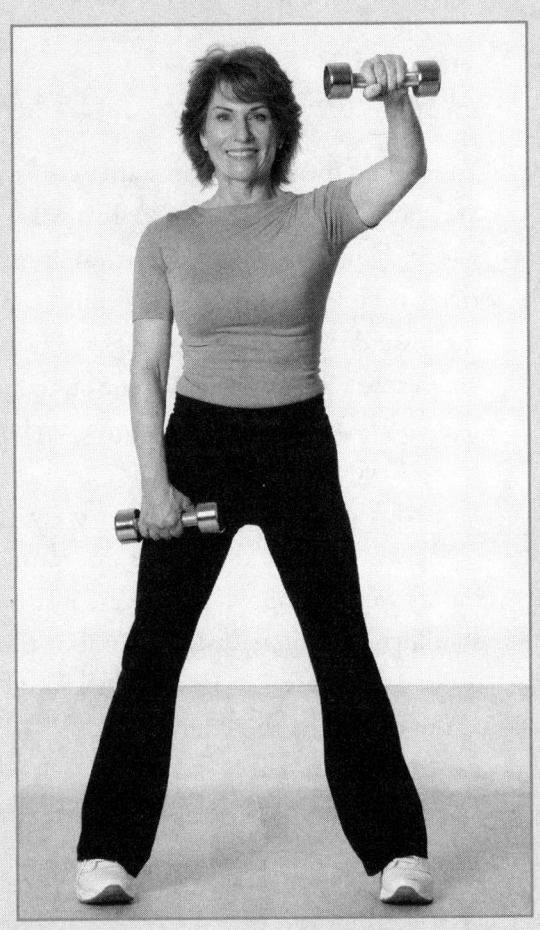

②

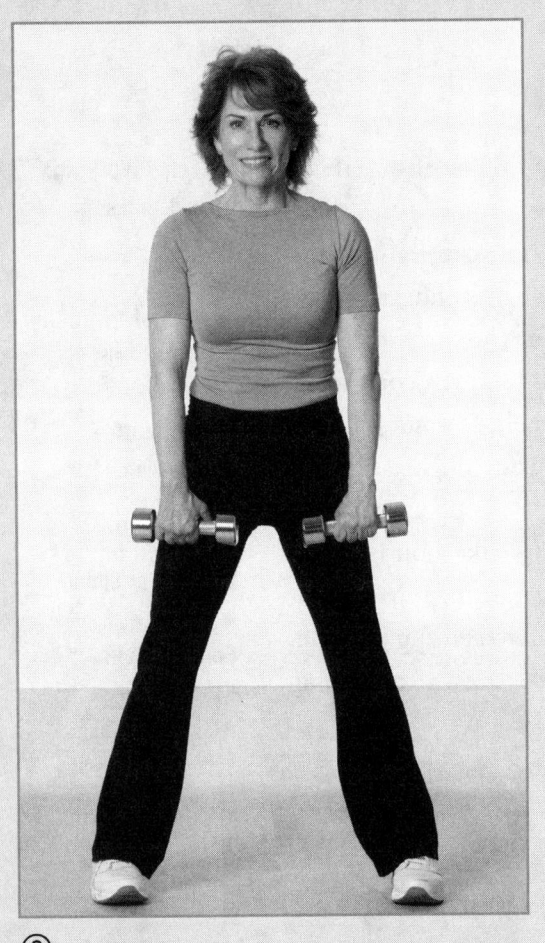

①

One-Arm Front Delt Lifts Using Dumbbells

EXECUTION

Stand with your feet planted firmly on the ground, a little wider than hip-distance apart, abdominal muscles tightly contracted. Hold a dumbbell firmly in each hand, placed in front of your thighs and with your fingers facing toward your body. Maintain a slight 5-degree bend in your elbow.

Slowly raise one dumbbell straight out in front of you, feeling a contraction in the front of your shoulder. Stop when your arm is just about even with your forehead. As you release the dumbbell down to starting position, do so slowly, resisting against gravity and feel a strong lengthening at the top of the shoulder. Do not rest between arms, but immediately repeat the One-Arm Front Delt Lift using the other arm.

Muscles Working:
Front of Shoulders
(Anterior Deltoid)

Degree of Difficulty:
One Dumbbell

Equipment:
Dumbbells

Body Position:
Standing or Sitting

Form Watch:
Keep your neck and shoulders relaxed, focusing your concentration on the muscles right in the front of your shoulder.

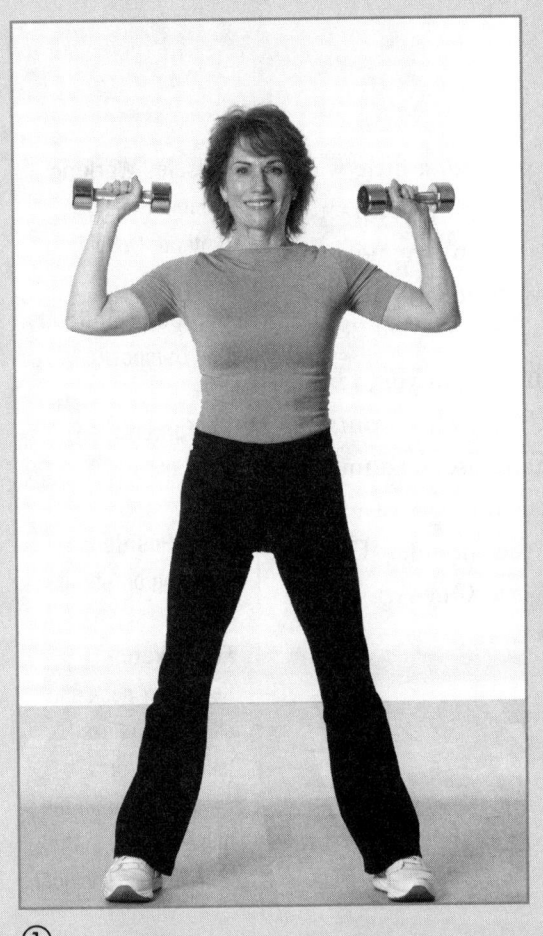

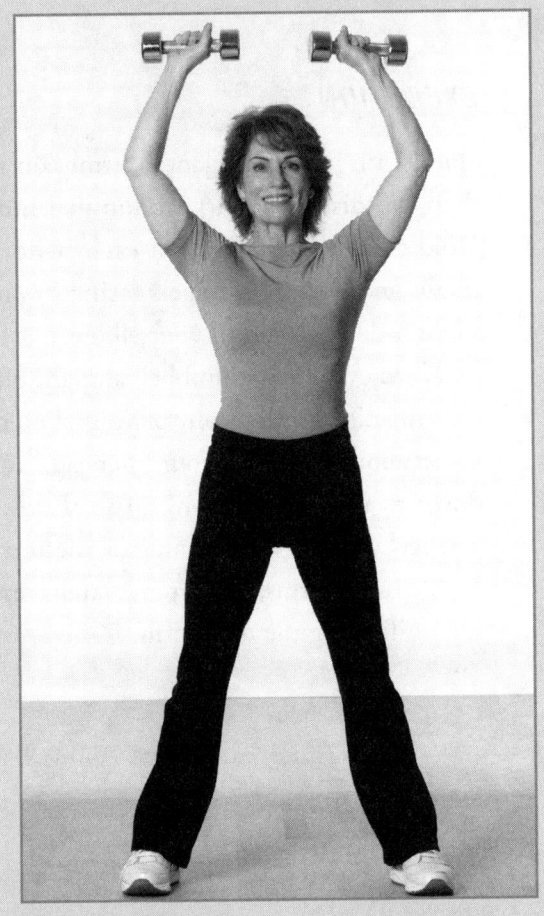

① ②

Overhead Presses Using Dumbbells

EXECUTION

You can do Overhead Presses either standing or sitting. If you are standing, plant your feet firmly on the ground, a little wider than hip-distance apart, abdominal muscles tightly contracted. If you are seated, sit up tall, spine straight, abdominals contracted. It is best to sit in a chair without a cushion to give your body stability. You can do these in the gym seated on a bench with the back inclined, so you can rest your spine against it.

Holding the dumbbells evenly-balanced in your hands with your fingertips facing outward, bring them up so they are just above your shoulders. From this position, raise your arms up slowly, bringing the dumbbells over the top of your head until the ends almost come together.

Slowly release the dumbbells to starting position, controlling the downward motion by contracting the muscles and resisting against the pull of gravity.

Muscles Working:
Top of Shoulders
(Lateral Deltoid)

Degree of Difficulty:
Two Dumbbells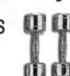

Equipment:
Dumbbells

Body Position:
Standing or Sitting

Form Watch:
Keep your neck relaxed and protect your back by maintaining a strong contraction in your abdominal muscles.

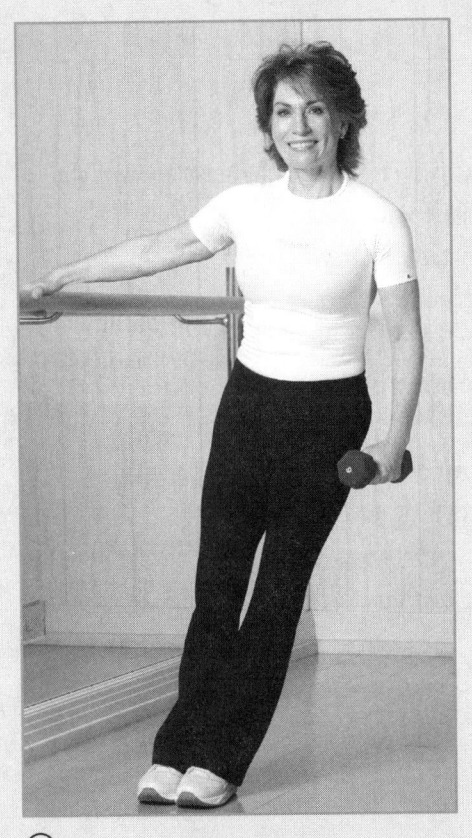 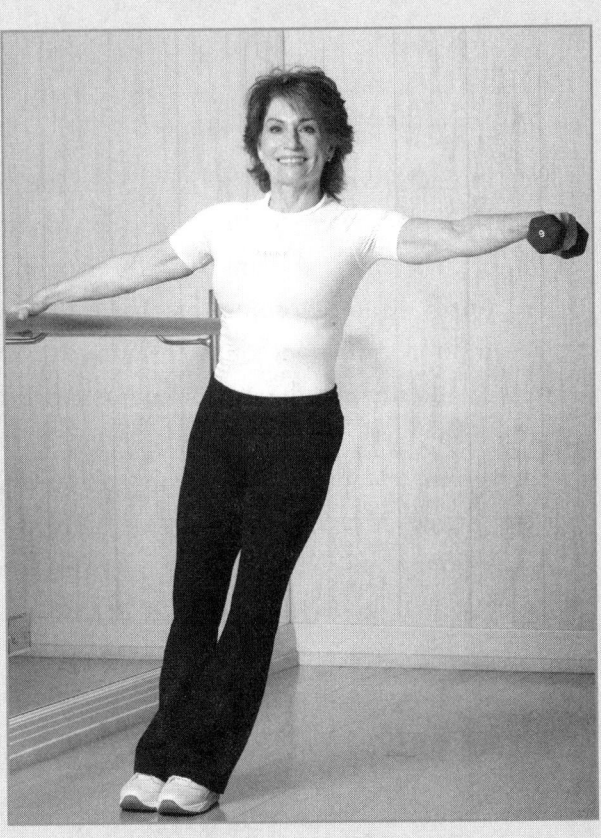

① ②

Angled One-Arm Side Raises

EXECUTION

Stand by the side of a stationary object, either a ballet barre, the frame of a piece of equipment in the gym, or other secured object. Hold a dumbbell in your work hand, evenly balanced with your fingertips facing toward your thighs. Position your body so your feet are closer to the object you are holding onto and your torso is slanted away from it. This shifts the force of gravity into your working arm.

Lift the dumbbell out to the side until it is just about even with the top of your shoulder. Maintain a slight bend in your elbow and keep your abdominal muscles and your buttocks muscles (glutes) tightly contracted to keep your posture in alignment.

Resisting against the natural force of gravity, slowly lower the dumbbell to starting position by the side of your thigh.

Muscles Working:
Top of Shoulders
(Lateral Deltoid)

Degree of Difficulty:
Two Dumbbells

Equipment:
Dumbbells

Body Position:
Standing

Form Watch:
In the slanted position, maintain a straight spine and keep a slight bend at the knee joint.

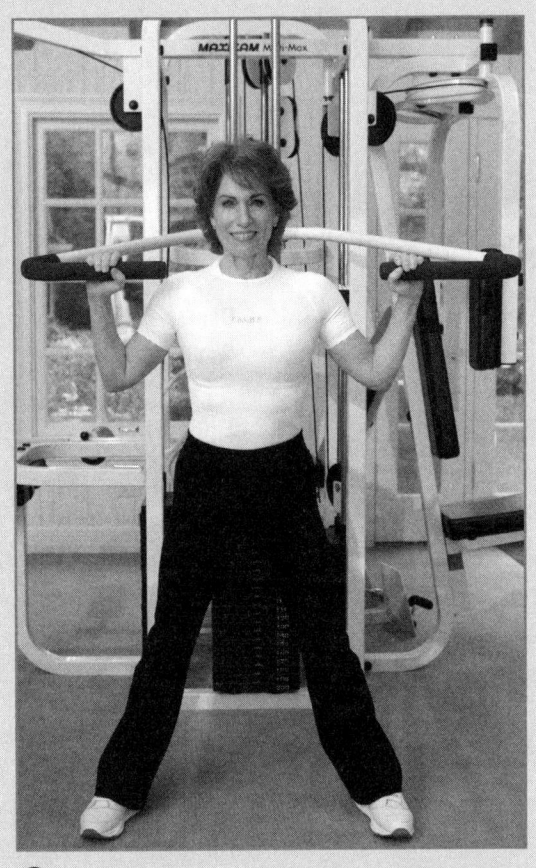

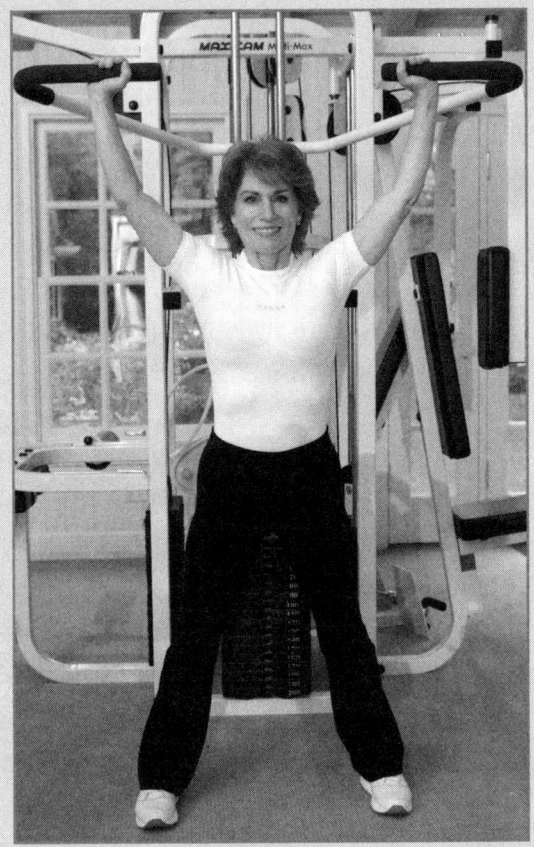

①   ②

Shoulder Press Machine

EXECUTION

Standing in front of the machine, align the arm levers so they are just above the top of your shoulders. Plant your feet firmly on the ground, wider than hip-distance apart, and contract your abdominal muscles.

Gripping the handles so your fingertips are facing forward, slowly lift up the machine until your arms are almost, but not completely, straight. You want to maintain a slight bend at the elbow joints.

As you lower the lever arm back to starting position, do so slowly, feeling a lengthening right in the top of the shoulders. Resist against the gravitational pull of the machine by keeping your deltoid muscles contracted.

Muscles Working:
Top of Shoulders
(Lateral Deltoid)

Degree of Difficulty:
Two Dumbbells

Equipment:
Shoulder Press
Machine

Body Position:
Standing

Form Watch:
Keep your neck and shoulders relaxed and in neutral position throughout the entire movement.

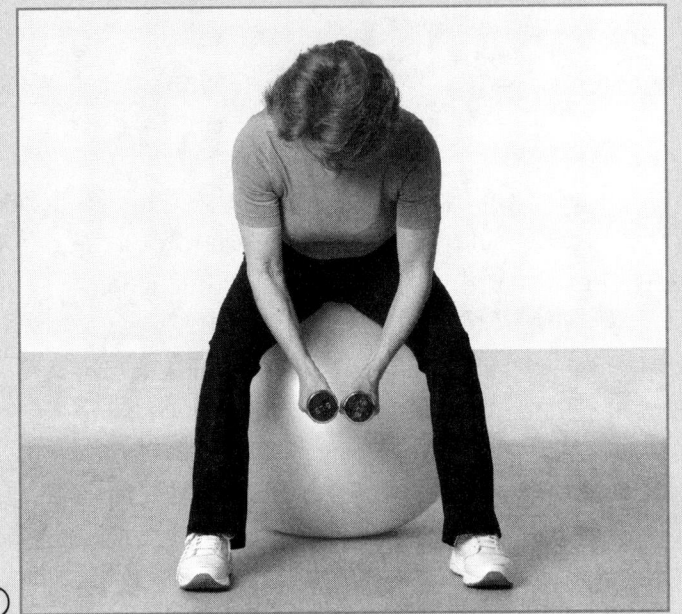

①

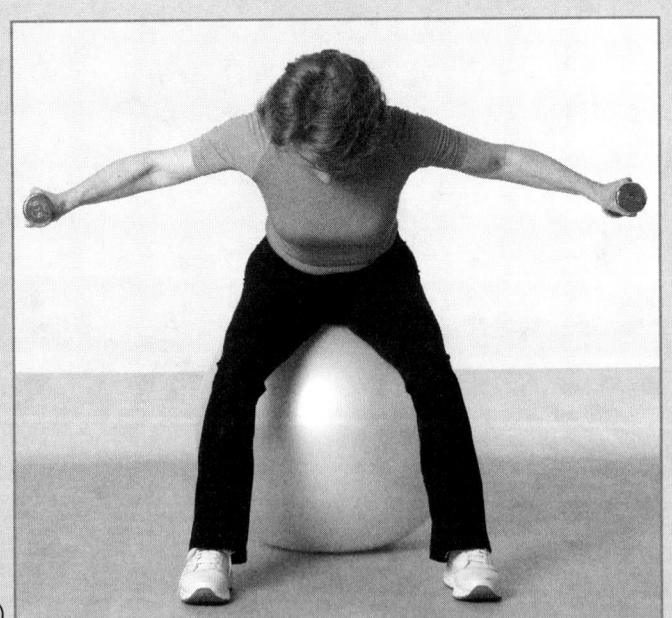

②

Reverse Flyes on Ball Using Dumbbells

EXECUTION

Sit on an exercise ball with your feet firmly planted on the ground and your abdominals tightly contracted. Good form is essential in order to keep the ball steady underneath you.

Bend over at the waist so your torso is almost parallel to the floor. Start with the dumbbells hanging in front of you, between your legs and parallel to one another. Slowly bring the dumbbells out to the sides until you feel a contraction in the back of your shoulder. Keep a slight bend in your elbow as you raise up your arms. Bring your arms up until you feel a squeeze between your shoulder blades, then slowly return your arms to starting position, with a controlled motion, resisting against gravity.

Muscles Working:
Back of Shoulders
(Posterior Deltoid)

Degree of Difficulty:
Three Dumbbells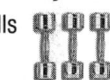

Equipment:
Dumbbells and
Exercise Ball

Body Position:
Seated

Form Watch:
Keep your head in alignment with your spine and your abdominals contracted the entire time.

Side Lateral Arm Raises

Muscles Working:
Top of Shoulders
(Deltoids)

Degree of Difficulty:
One Dumbbell

Equipment:
None Required

Body Position:
Seated or Standing

Form Watch:
If standing, bend
slightly forward. If
seated, give your
arms enough room to
come out all the way
to the sides of your
body.

EXECUTION

If you are standing, place your feet shoulder-width apart to create a solid base, keep your abdominals contracted the entire time. If you are seated, sit at the edge of a sturdy chair without arms or a bench so you can bring your arms out to the side freely. Place your fists in front of your pelvic bone. Maintain a slight bend in your elbow. Your hands are forming fists with the insides of your wrists facing each other. Slowly extend your arms out to the sides like the wings of a bird about to take flight. Bring them up until they end up just level with your shoulders. Keep your neck relaxed. Return arms slowly to starting position in front of the pelvic bone.

Overhead Shoulder Presses

EXECUTION

You can do Overhead Shoulder Presses either seated or standing. If standing, place your feet shoulder-width apart. If seated, sit up straight without resting your back on the chair. Keep abdominals contracted. Bring your hands up so they are slightly above but parallel to your shoulders, and your elbows are in a 90-degree angle. Your hands are in a closed-fist position. Move your arms up, in a half circle, above your head so in the end position your hands meet above your head with your wrists facing forward. At the top position, arms are not completely straight but maintain a soft bend in your elbows. As you bring your arms back to starting position, keep a wide arch in your arms so your arms do not come in too close to your head. Do not rush either the upward or downward movements. (See photo on page 146 as an example of proper form and technique for this exercise.)

Muscles Working:
Shoulders (Deltoids)

Degree of Difficulty:
One Dumbbell

Equipment:
None Required

Body Position:
Seated or Standing

Form Watch:
Keep your neck and shoulders tension free.

Reverse Flyes

Equipment-Free Exercises

Muscles Working:
Shoulders (Rear Deltoids)

Degree of Difficulty:
One Dumbbell

Equipment:
None Required

Body Position:
Standing or Seated

Form Watch:
Keep your arms and upper body contracted, and feel the squeeze in the back of the shoulders and shoulder blades.

EXECUTION

In standing position, place your feet shoulder-width apart to create a solid base. Contract your abdominals. Bend forward slightly at the waist, enough so your torso is facing toward the floor. If you are seated, sit at the edge of a sturdy chair without arms or a bench so you are able to bring your arms out behind you freely. Lean your torso forward slightly so you're bending at the waist. Your arms are hanging down, so your hands are in front of your thighs. Your hands are forming fists with your fingers facing one another. From starting position, leaning slightly forward at the waist, bring your arms out behind your. Your arms should not be completely straight but maintain a slight bend in the elbow joint. Bring your arms up just level with your shoulders. You will feel the contraction in the back of your shoulders and upper back. Lower your arms to starting position without rushing the movement. (See photo on page 152 as an example of proper form and technique for this exercise.)

Hard Core

Flatter "Abs" and Stronger "Back" Forever More

Nothing is unthinkable, nothing impossible to the balanced person . . .

LEWIS MUMFORD

I was in the lady's restroom of a trendy Sunset Boulevard restaurant with my friend, Jennifer, one evening when she came storming out of the stall, her shirt yanked up under her bra, exposing her mid-section, screaming at me, "You're a fitness expert! What is this and how the hell do I get rid of it?" Jennifer is tall and slim (for the most part), except for some noticeable midriff adiposity.

"Well," I said starting off slowly and backing toward the exit door because I knew she wasn't going to be thrilled with what I was about to say, ". . . now don't shoot the messenger, that is middle age spread."

"What?! I'm thin. I walk three or four times a week! Why do I have middle age spread?"

"Ah, well," and I tried to break the news as softly as possible, "you're middle aged." Luckily, the bar of soap hit the restroom door before it came crashing down in front of my feet.

When we returned to our table for coffee, I said to Jenny seriously, "Listen, the spread around your middle is not an inevitable part of the aging process, honestly. It's just that your metabolism has slowed down. And in menopausal women, when that happens the fat often accumulates around the middle."

"Well, I don't like it. Can I get rid off it?"

"Yes. With the correct exercises and doing them properly, an honest commitment to your program and consistency, you can definitely strengthen and trim the mid body."

Jennifer's desire to reduce her middle body fat is not in vanity's name only. Central body fat not only prevents us from buttoning our pants, it also has some dangerous metabolic side effects. A number of studies support findings that implicate mid-body fat with an increase in coronary heart disease (CHD). An article in the *American Journal of Epidemiology*, on the association between central obesity and heart disease and mortality in postmenopausal women, reported, ". . . numerous studies have documented that abdominal obesity, compared with overall adiposity as estimated by body mass index (BMI), is more strongly associated with both CHD risk factors and CHD events."

The pattern of body fat distribution is a valuable predictor of health-related problems. Trunk or abdominal fat is directly correlated to increased risk for type 2 diabetes, the fastest growing disease in the world today, elevated blood lipids, high blood pressure and heart disease. Some studies link mid-body fat to colon cancer, breast and uterine cancer.

Additionally, mid-body fat shifts our center of gravity, which increases our risk for back problems related to a form of poor posture called lordosis. It is commonly referred to as being "swaybacked." A swaybacked posture is an extreme curve between the ribs of the lumbar region and the pelvis resulting in your stomach sticking out too far in front of you and your buttocks stick out too far behind.

YOUR WAIST—HIP RATIO

As stated earlier, your waist circumference has been strongly associated with heart disease and mortality rates, especially in postmenopausal women. It seems to be the speed at which weight is gained and location of the fat deposits that causes the most concern.

A very easy method for determining your risk for disease related to mid-body fat is measuring your waist-hip ratio. You simply measure the circumference of your waist divided by the circumference of the hips. For instance, if your waist is 27 and your hips are 36 you would divide 27 by 36 = 0.75.

Women should be below 0.82
Men should be below 0.94

Given the serious consequences of central body fat and its health implications, it is especially vital for menopausal women to devote concentrated effort to strengthening the abdominal area as well as the back areas in something called Total Core Strengthening. While you can't "spot reduce," you can definitely strengthen and firm your abdominal area. You will need a consistent program of aerobic exercise, to help you burn fat and lose weight all over. Then, the Core exercises described in this Strategy will help you tighten and condense your body's mid-area for a slimmer, healthier body composition.

CORE ANATOMY

Your core is your body's center of gravity. It is comprised of the muscles in your pelvis, lower back, hips, and abdominal area. When these muscles are strong and work harmoniously, they help stabilize and protect your spine for movements as elementary as walking and as rigorous as a tennis match with Anna Kournikova. The goal is to strengthen all the core muscles equally, so that they work synergistically to provide stabilization. Should one muscle group become too powerful there is an inequitable demand on that muscle and you run the risk of injury. It can also result in poor posture, which can cause chronic discomfort, height loss throughout the aging process, and limited mobility. Following is a brief description of the muscles comprising the core structure.

THE ABDOMINAL MUSCLES

Your abdominal area is comprised of four different muscles. This is important to know because we often erroneously think of our mid-region as one big muscle. In order to train the muscles correctly, each must be isolated and worked separately or in concert with co-contracting muscles for maximum results.

1. Rectus abdominis: This muscle is the one you normally think of as your "abs" because it is located in the mid-section of your abdominal area and you can feel it when you touch your center. It starts at the crest of the pubic bone and attaches at the fifth, sixth, and seventh ribs and the xiphoid process, which is that little bone between your breasts. The rectus (which means straight) helps control the curvature of the lower spine by controlling the angle of the pelvis. It is responsible for helping you flex forward as well as side-to-side.

2. External obliques: If you touch the sides of your midriff, you can feel the external oblique muscles. These muscles are responsible for lumbar flexion, a bowing move, for instance, in case you meet the Queen of England. The right side externals allow you to flex to the right and help you rotate to the left. And, of course, the left externals do the opposite. Additionally, the left external oblique is the one strongly engaged and contracted when doing sits-ups when the torso rotates to the right and the right externals are deeply contracted when the torso twists to the left.

3. Internal obliques: These bi-lateral muscles run diagonally in the opposite direction to that of the external obliques. While doing sits up with a twisting action touching the right elbow to the left knee, the right external obliques and the left internal obliques rotate simultaneously serving as synergistic muscles to help the rectus in flexing the torso to make the motion complete and vice versa.

4. Transversus abdominis: You can't feel this muscle, but it is located in the mid-section of your abdominal area, starting from the cartilage of the lower six ribs, inserting at the top of the pubic bone. It serves almost like a girdle around your mid-section. It is the major player in helping hold your abdominals flat. Its main action is forced expiration by contracting the abdominal wall inward. One of the best ways to work it is with an isometric contraction, pulling it back toward the spine.

THE BACK MUSCLES

The erector spinae muscle is the largest muscle mass of the back. It lies in the intermediate layer of the intrinsic back muscles and is actually divided into three longitudinal muscle columns—the iliocostalis, longissimus, and the spinalis—that run parallel to the spine. It is responsible for back extension, for instance when you stretch your back while yawning, and lateral (side) flexion of the spine, moving side to side.

In this Strategy I give you twelve exercises specifically targeted to help with your entire core strengthening by focusing attention on both the abdominals and the erector spinae muscle groups.

I also include in this Strategy two exercises, Pelvic Tilts and Kegels, which work the muscles around the pelvic floor. Although these muscles are not are not part of your core structure, I included them here because through childbirth and the aging process these muscles become weaker, which can result in pain around the vaginal area and a condition referred to as stress incontinence.

BODY PRESERVING EXERCISES—CORE

1 Ball Crunches
2 Lateral Side Drops on Exercise Ball
3 Quadruped Using Ankle Weights
4 Crunches on Flat Bench Using Resistance Ball
5 Reverse Leg Lifts Using Ankle Weights
6 Back Extensions on Exercise Ball

Equipment-Free Body Preserving Core and Pelvic Exercises:

7 Isometric Squeezes
8 Leg Lifts
9 Pelvic Tilts
10 Sitting Leg Lifts
11 Classic Crunches
12 Kegels
13 Cycle Rotations
14 Plank and Modified Plank

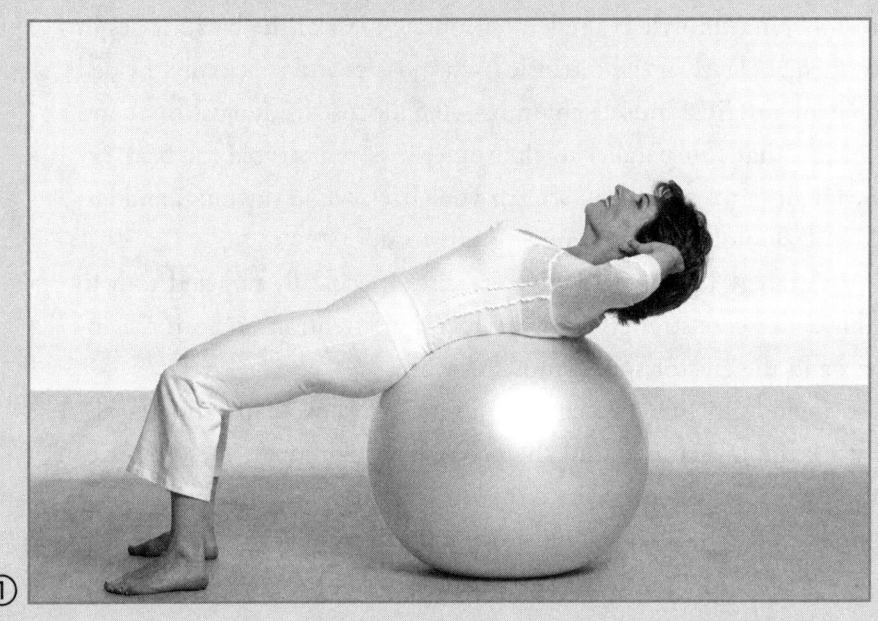

①

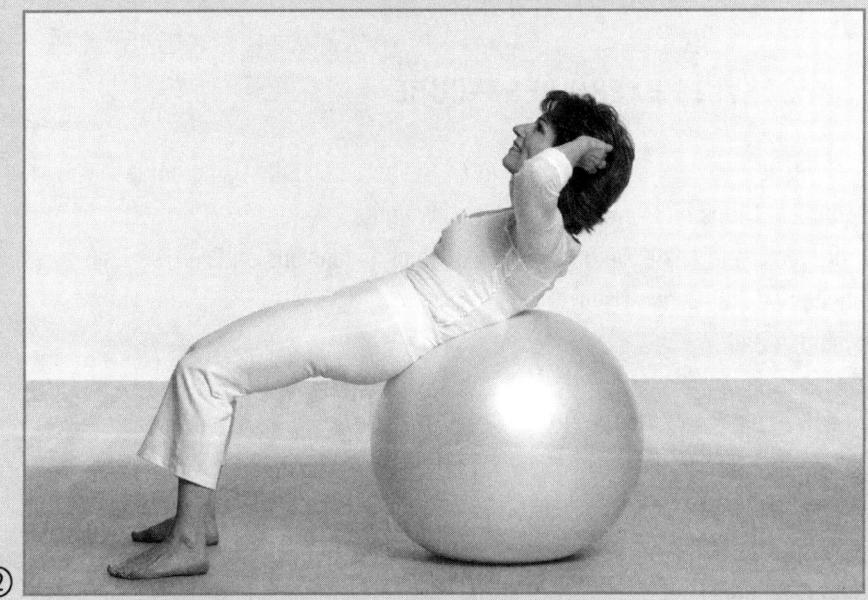

②

Ball Crunches

EXECUTION

If you don't own an exercise ball, it's a great and inexpensive work-out accessory that is very versatile for use with many different exercises. They cost anywhere from twenty-five dollars to as much as fifty or sixty dollars. Price is based on the size of the ball. The size of the ball that is correct for you is based on your height. Following is a guideline to help you make the correct selection:

Height:	Ball Size:
5 feet to 5'7"	55 cm
5'7" to 6'2"	65 cm

Only do this exercise if you feel very secure and comfortable on the ball and if you have no trouble leaning backward.

Position yourself on the ball so you're evenly balanced. Hands are at the sides or behind your head with elbows pointed out-wards. In this position, eyes looking up at the ceiling, chest open, lift your torso up off the ball as far as you can, feeling a squeeze in the upper abdominals.

Muscles Working:
Upper Abs (Rectus Abdominis)

Degree of Difficulty:
One Dumbbell

Equipment:
Exercise Ball

Body Position:
Lying

Form Watch:
Don't pull on your neck. The movements should be done slowly.

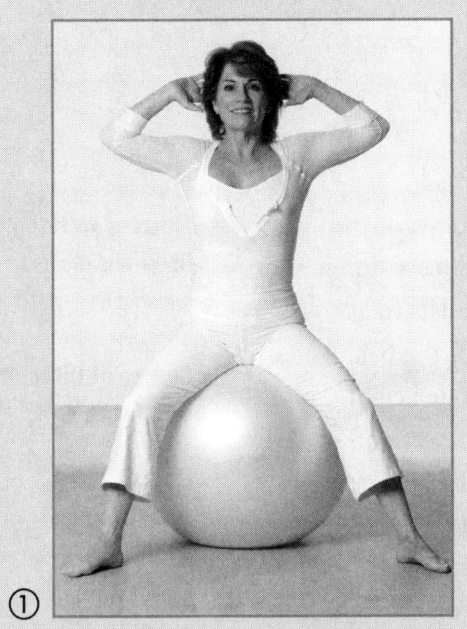

①

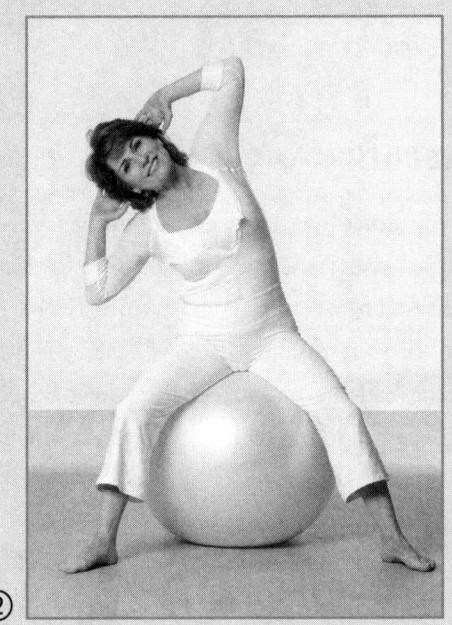

②

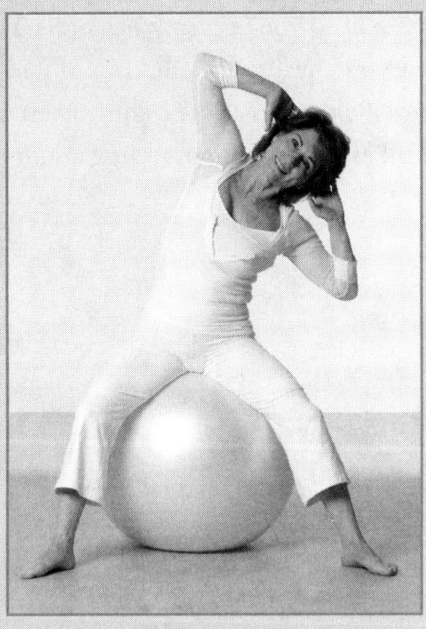

③

Lateral Side Drops on Exercise Ball

EXECUTION

Make certain you feel comfortable and safe while sitting on the ball. Place feet firmly on the floor. To help stabilize your body while you're seated on the ball, isometrically squeeze your abdominals. Now place your hands behind your head with elbows pointed outwards. Leading with your elbow, slowly drop to the right. You will feel a gentle stretch on the left. Now come up to starting position and slowly drop to the left and feel the stretch on the right.

Muscles Working:
Sides of the Abdominals (Internal, External Obliques)

Degree of Difficulty:
One Dumbbell

Equipment:
Exercise Ball

Body Position:
Seated

Form Watch:
Keep your abs contracted throughout the entire exercise.

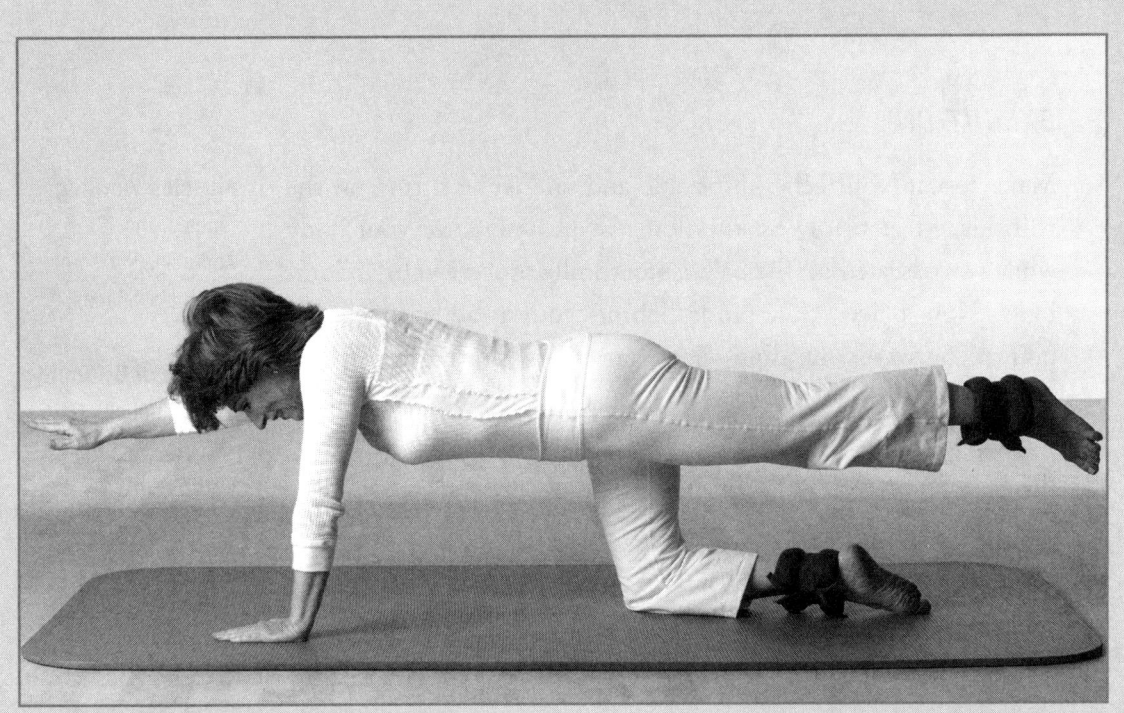

Quadruped Using Ankle Weights

EXECUTION

The starting position for this exercise is on hands and knees. Wrap the weights around your ankles so they are secure and won't shift around on your leg. Isometrically contracting your abdominals, raise one hand and the opposite leg off the floor lifting it straight out behind you. Hold this position, squeezing the buttocks and maintaining a tight contraction in the abdominals, for a count of five seconds and repeat on the other side.

Muscle Working:
Abdominals, Muscles of the Back and Buttocks (Transversus Abdominis, Erector Spinae, Gluteus Medius)

Equipment:
Ankle Weights

Degree of Difficulty:
Two Dumbbells

Body Position:
Hands and Knees

Form Watch:
Contracting the abdominal muscles throughout the exercise will help you maintain your balance and train you to isolate these muscles. This is a great lower back strengthening exercise!

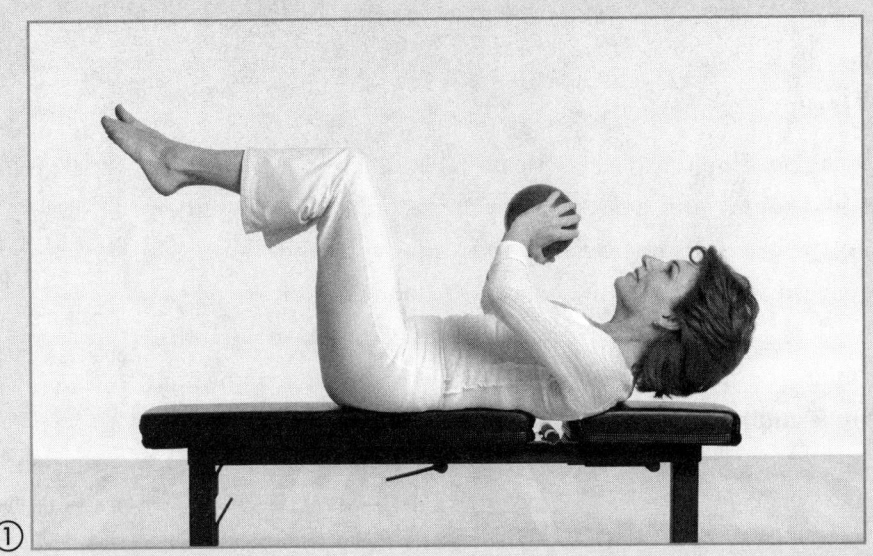

①

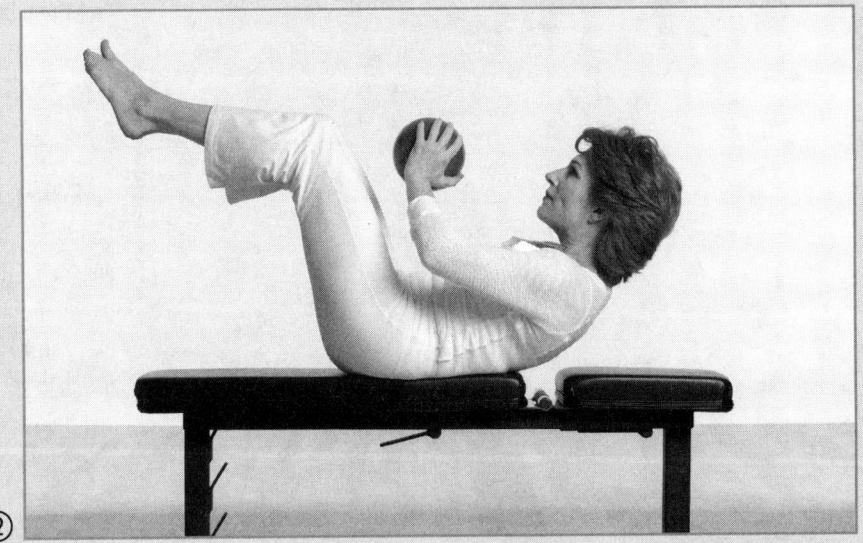

②

Crunches on Flat Bench Using Resistance Ball

EXECUTION

Lie on an exercise bench and place your feet together and bring your legs up so your knees are at a 90-degree angle.

Holding a weighted exercise ball between your hands, isometrically squeeze the abdominals, so you can feel the muscles pulling towards your spine. With your eyes facing towards the ceiling, lift your shoulders up slightly off the bench. That is your starting and ending position. Then, in one integrated movement, lift up your torso and curve it toward your legs. On the release back toward the bench, lower your back but do not let the shoulders touch down on the bench.

Muscle Working:
Upper Abdominals
(Rectus Abdominis)

Degree of Difficulty:
Two Dumbbells

Equipment:
Flat Bench and
Weighted Exercise Ball

Position:
Lying

Form Watch:
Do not release the contraction in your abdominal muscles. They remain tightly squeezed the entire time, and don't forget to breathe.

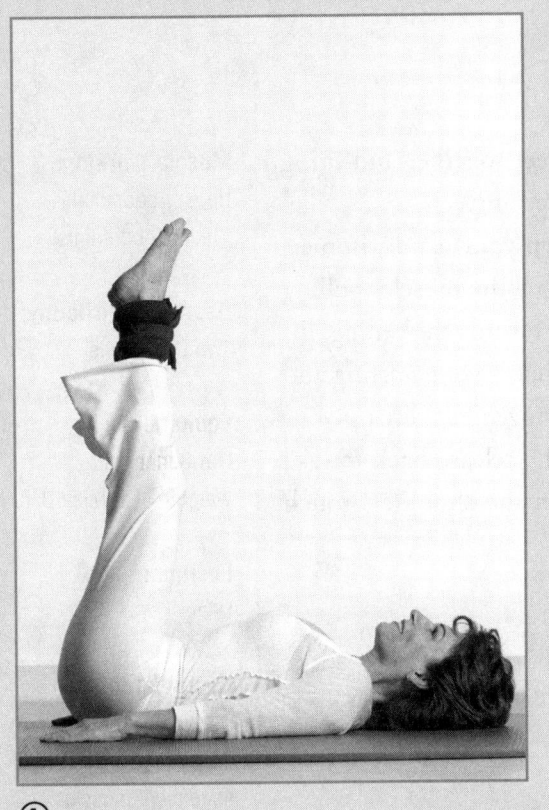

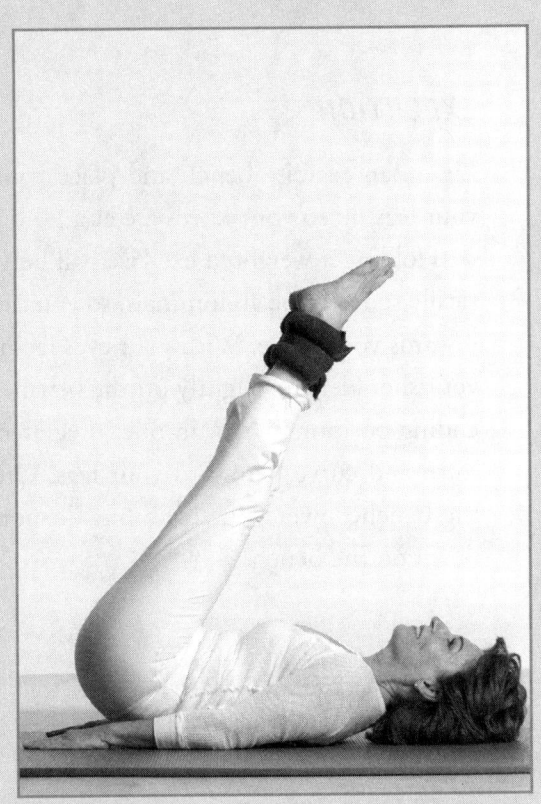

①   ②

Reverse Leg Lifts Using Ankle Weights

EXECUTION

You can do these either on a flat bench or on the floor. If you are on a flat bench, place your buttocks toward the edge of the bench so your legs can swing freely and firmly grip the sides of the bench with your hands. If you are on the floor, place your hands by your sides. Attach ankle weights securely so they don't shift as you move.

Place your legs and feet together maintaining a slight bend in your knees. Keeping your legs together, contract your abdominal muscles, lift up your buttocks, and flex your hips so your legs are moving toward your chest. Control the move by keeping your abdominal muscles tightly contracted.

As you bring your legs back to starting position, feel a strong lengthening of the lower abdominals without letting your lower back arch up off the floor or bench.

Muscles Working:
Lower Abdominals
(Lower Rectus
Abdominis)

Degree of Difficulty:
Three Dumbbells

Equipment:
Ankle Weights

Body Position:
Lying

Form Watch:
Do not let the legs
"swing" toward the
chest, but carefully
control the motion by
contracting the
abdominal muscles.

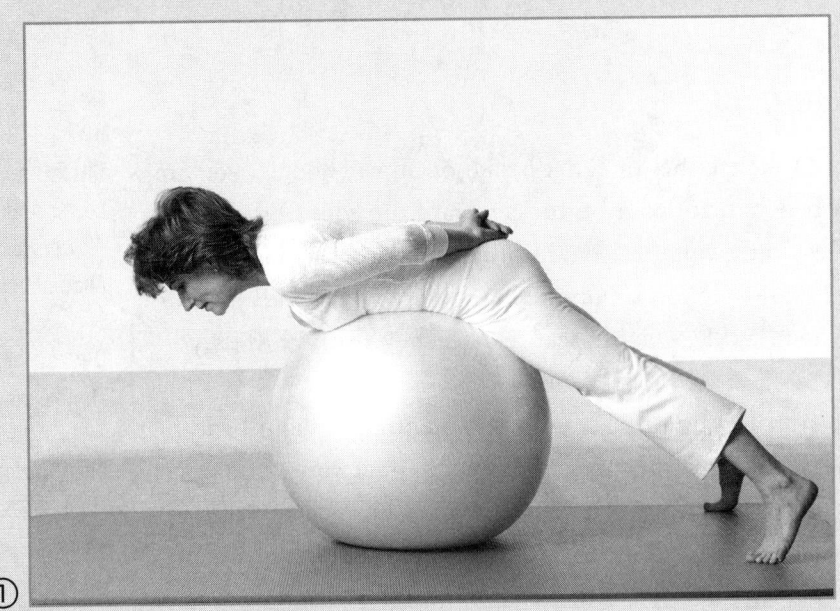

①

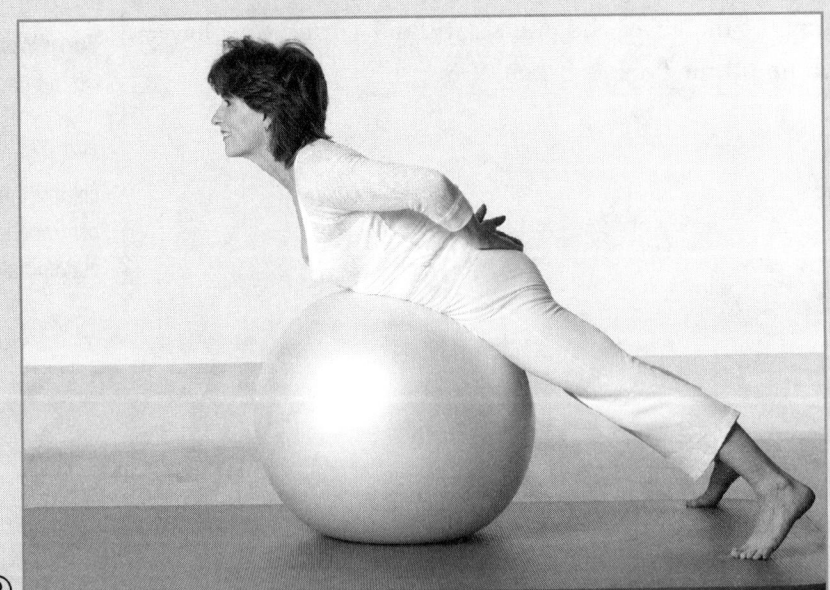

②

Back Extensions on Exercise Ball

EXECUTION

Carefully place your body over an exercise ball so your torso is resting comfortably over the ball. Place your feet on the ground, wide enough apart so you feel secure on the ball. You can place your hands either folded, resting on the small of your back, or straight out in front of you, which is a little more challenging, so only do this when you're feeling totally comfortable on the ball.

From starting position, contract your gluteal muscles and slowly lift your torso up off the ball as far back as you can. You will feel a contraction at the top of your glutes and a squeeze in your lower back. Hold the squeeze and then slowly return to starting position.

Muscle Working:
Muscles of the Back and Buttocks (Erector Spinae, Gluteals)

Equipment:
Exercise Ball

Degree of Difficulty:
Three Dumbbells

Body Position:
Prone Position Over Ball

Form Watch:
Keep your head in alignment with a straight spine and your abdominal muscles contracted the entire time.

Isometric Squeezes

Muscles Working:
Abdominals (Rectus and Trasversus)

Degree of Difficulty:
One Dumbbell

Equipment:
None Required

Body Position:
Seated, standing, or lying down

Form Watch:
As you pull in your abdominal muscles, do not hold your breath, but breathe normally throughout the contraction without releasing the tight contraction.

EXECUTION

Isometric squeezes can be done anywhere, any place, seated, standing, or lying down. One way to practice what an isometric contraction feels like is to release a little cough. Place your hand on your abdominals and you will feel them tightening as your ribcage lifts slightly. That is the feel of the isometric squeeze. It is very important when you pull in your abdominals that you don't forget to breath. Also, this should be the first exercise you do before performing any of the other abdominal exercises as well as most all exercises you do, whether seated, standing, or lying.

Leg Lifts

EXECUTION

Sit on the floor and place your hands behind you. You are leaning back slightly on your hands. Place your legs and feet together maintaining a slight bend in your knees. Contracting your abdominal muscles, lift your legs about an inch off the floor. From this position lift up your legs higher, bringing your knees toward your chest and your chest toward your knees in a jack-knife action.

Muscles Working:
Lower Abdominals
(Lower Rectus
Abdominis)

Degree of Difficulty:
Three Dumbbells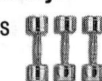

Equipment:
None Required

Body Position:
Sitting

Form Watch:
As you lower your legs, bring them down far enough so you feel a strong lengthening of the lower abdominals.

Pelvic Tilts

Muscle Working:
Pelvic Floor Muscles
and Lower Abdominals
(Lower Rectus)

Degree of Difficulty:
One Dumbbell

Equipment:
None Required

Body Position:
Lying on the Ground,
Knees Bent.

Form Watch:
Don't over-arch or lift
your buttocks so far
off the ground that
you are putting too
much pressure on
your neck and
shoulders.

EXECUTION

Lie flat on the floor, knees bent. In this position, lift your buttocks off the ground but do not lift up so high your back comes off the floor. In this position, perform a series of mini contractions and releases by squeezing the buttocks together.

Sitting Leg Lifts

EXECUTION

Do these Sitting Leg Lifts on a very stable chair or workout bench. From an upright seated position, place your hands at your sides, gripping the chair or bench so your body is angled slightly backward. Before lifting the legs, make certain to tightly squeeze the abdominal muscles. While the abs are held tightly, with your legs together, thighs touching, lift your legs up high enough so the back of your legs lift off the chair or bench. You will feel the movement in your lower and middle abdominals.

Muscles Working:
Lower Abdominals
(Lower Rectus)

Degree of Difficulty:
One Dumbbell

Equipment:
None Required

Body Position:
Sitting

Form Watch:
Keep your abdominal muscles squeezed tightly the entire time and don't let your feet touch the ground.

Classic Crunches

Muscle Working:
Upper Abdominals
(Rectus Abdominis)

Degree of Difficulty:
One Dumbbell

Equipment:
None Required

Position:
Lying

Form Watch:
When you lift up, lead
with your chest and
make sure not to pull
on your neck.

EXECUTION

Lie on the floor with your knees bent and your feet placed about 15 inches in front of your body, creating a triangular space.

Gently rest your hands behind your head without pulling on your neck. Before performing the "crunch action," isometrically squeeze the abdominals, so you can feel the muscles pulling towards your spine. Now with eyes facing towards the ceiling, head and neck in neutral position, in one integrated movement lift up into the crunch, squeezing the rectus muscle. On the release back toward the floor, lower your back but do not let the shoulders touch the floor. And don't forget to breathe!

Kegel Exercises

EXECUTION

Throughout the aging process many women, as well as some men, suffer from stress urinary incontenence because of weaked pelvic floor muscles. The symptom includes involuntary loss of urine during physical exertion with increased intraabdominal pressure, such as with coughing, sneezing, laughing, exercise, lifting, or sitting. The urine loss is usually not a large amount but the frequency with which it occurs may require wearing a pad constantly to avoid embarrassment. Urinary incontinence has been reported to affect 35% of American women over 50 years of age and almost 15% have leakage on a daily basis. When performed properly and consistently, Kegel exercises have been shown to be 50–80% effective in improving stress urinary continence.

Kegel exercises can be performed any time and any place. Many women perfer performing the exercises while lying down or sitting in a chair. After 4 to 6 weeks, most people notice some improvement. It may take as long as 3 months to see a significant change.

Several techniques help will help you identify the correct muscles. One approach is to sit on the toilet and start to urinate. Try to stop the flow of urine midstream by contracting your pelvic floor muscles. Repeat this action several times until you become familiar with the feel of contracting the correct group of muscles. Do not contract your abdominal, thigh, or buttock muscles while performing the exercise.

Equipment-Free Exercises

Muscles Working:
Pelvic Floor Muscles

Degree of Difficulty:
One Dumbbell

Equipment:
None Required

Body Position:
Lying Down, Seated, or Standing

Form Watch:
Don't hold your breath while performing the contractions. If you feel any discomfort in your abdomen or back you are probably not doing the Kegel exercises properly. Just relax and concentrate on squeezing the pelvic floor muscles.

Kegel Exercises (continued)

**Equipment-Free
Exercises**

Muscles Working:
Pelvic Floor Muscles

Degree of Difficulty:
One Dumbbell

Equipment:
None Required

Body Position:
Lying Down, Seated,
or Standing

Form Watch:
Don't hold your breath
while performing the
contractions. If you
feel any discomfort in
your abdomen or back
you are probably not
doing the Kegel
exercises properly.
Just relax and
concentrate on
squeezing the pelvic
floor muscles.

Another approach to help you identify the correct muscle group is to insert a finger into the vagina. Try to tighten the muscles around your finger as if holding back urine. The abdominal and thigh muscles should remain relaxed.

Perform pelvic floor exercises by first emptying your bladder. Squeeze the pelvic floor muscles and hold for a count of 10 and then release. Repeat the squeeze-and-release action 10 times, three times a day.

Because no one can see what you are doing, you can even do these exercises while waiting in line at the supermarket or even driving your car!

Cycle Rotations

EXECUTION

Cycle Rotations are the best way to work both the upper and lower abdominal muscles at the same time. The form mimics the movement your legs would make while riding a bicycle but, of course, you are not on a bicycle but lying on the floor.

Lying on your back, bring your legs up so that your knees are at a 90-degree angle to your body. Lift your shoulders off the ground and place your hands behind your head with your elbows pointing outward. This is your starting position. Your shoulders never touch the ground while doing this exercise.

Contracting your abdominals tightly, from this position you twist one elbow toward the opposite knee as you simultaneously bring the knee toward the elbow so they meet about mid body. Then repeat the same action on the other side, twisting and bringing the opposite elbow toward the opposite knee. Keep a steady breathing pattern with each rotation.

Muscle Working:
Upper and Sides of the Abdominals (Rectus, Internal and External Obliques)

Degree of Difficulty:
Two Dumbbells

Equipment:
None Required

Position:
Lying

Form Watch:
Do not pull on your neck doing the cycle rotations. One way to prevent this is to place your hands more on the sides of your head rather than locked behind it.

Plank and Modified Plank

Muscle Working:
Abdominals, Core
(Transversus
Abdominis, Erector
Spinae, Gluteus
Medius)

Equipment:
None Required

Degree of Difficulty:
Two Dumbbells or
Three Dumbbells

Body Position:
Prone (face down) on
Hands and Feet

Form Watch:
Do not arch your back
or sink in the center.
Spine is straight.

EXECUTION

Plank is another exercise that really isolates and utilizes the abs. Resting your elbows on the ground, legs straight out behind you, lift your body up off the ground. You're balancing on your forearms and the toes of your feet. You can clasp your hands together, or have your arms parallel to one another. Isometrically contract the abdominal area and also squeeze the buttocks.

For Modified Plank, rest your knees on the ground, contract the abdominal muscles while squeezing the buttock muscles. Hold this position.

Stretching Your Body and Balancing Your Life

The Life Balancing Exercises®

The soul is the voice of the body's interests.

GEORGE SANTAYANA

"If you're not stretching, you're shrinking," I tell Liz. Liz is a fifty-five-year-old woman who recently retired from her career as the director of media relations for a *Fortune* 500 company. She is in good health, but over the years she has put on extra weight, lost physical strength and muscle tone, and feels generally weak and out of condition. She is over most of her menopausal symptoms but still suffers from disordered sleeping.

"I like to stretch," she says. "I know it is good for me, but I don't do it regularly because it seems like a waste of time and you've given me so many other exercises to do."

Poor overlooked stretching. It is the neglected second cousin to its two more famous exercise relatives, cardiovascular and strength training. But it is an essential member of the exercise family, and, as I tell Liz, "one that will serve you well throughout the aging process. Plus, it may help you sleep better."

According to a study conducted at the Fred Hutchinson Cancer Research Center in Seattle, Washington, "Both stretching and exercise interventions may improve sleep quality in sedentary, overweight, postmenopausal women. Increased fitness was associated with improvements in sleep."

Additionally, stretching regularly and correctly protects your ability to enjoy your activities of daily life. We can lose about fifty percent (or even more if sedentary) of our range of motion capabilities throughout the aging process if we aren't using our joints in their full range of motion. Inflexibility also results in joint stiffness and difficulty doing such normal activities as getting out of a car easily or bending down to pick up a golf ball or tennis ball pain free.

Moving fluidly without pain and stiffness is well worth the five to seven minutes a day a good and effective stretch exercise program will take.

WHAT HAPPENS WHEN WE STRETCH

When we stretch our muscles and tendons (the fibrous connective tissue that attaches muscles to bones) they lengthen. Surrounding our muscles are two highly sensitive receptors that monitor our stretching activities: muscle spindles and Golgi tendon organs. Muscle spindles are aligned parallel to the muscle fiber itself. When your muscle stretches, the spindles stretch as well, monitoring the amount of stretch you are placing on your muscle. If the stretch is perceived as dangerous, the components of the muscle spindles contract, stopping the stretch action and helping to prevent you from having an injury. The Golgi tendon organs are located in the tendons near where the muscle attaches. The Golgi tendon organs monitor the tension on your muscle. If they sense too much tension, they cause a reflex inhibition of the muscle, signaling it to relax thus protecting it and the tendon from injury caused by excessive load.

Stretching regularly and properly helps to re-educate these reflex mechanisms so the more you stretch, the more they sense a change in the amount of tension that is safe to place on a particular muscle.

SELF TEST—SIT AND REACH

Following is a simple but accurate test you can do at home to measure your forward flexion. You can do it by yourself but it may help to have a friend assist you with the reading (and possibly cheer you on!).

YOUR SIT AND REACH SCORE

Age	Inches Reached	Rating
40–49	< 10.5	Very Poor
	12.0–15.0	Poor
	16.5–18.0	Fair
	18.5–19.5	Good
	19.5–20.5	Excellent
	22 +	Superior
50–59	< 12.5	Very Poor
	12.5–15.0	Poor
	15.1–17.5	Fair
	17.6–18.0	Good
	18.5–20.0	Excellent
	23+	Superior
60+	< 9.2	Very Poor
	11.5–13.0	Poor
	13.5–15.5	Fair
	16.0–17.0	Good
	17.5–19.5	Excellent
	21+	Superior

Only do this test after a brief warm up, a five minute walk around the house or block, or in the middle of the day after you've moved around a bit or even have had a warm shower. Never conduct it on cold muscles or immediately upon waking up.

Place a yardstick on the floor with the 36-inch end placed against a wall. Take a piece of masking tape and place it across the yardstick at a right angle to the 15-inch mark.

Sit down, position yourself so that the yardstick is between your legs and your heels are up against the masking tape line. Your heels should be about 10 to 12 inches apart.

Now slowly reach forward with both hands, one can be placed on top of the other or both can be outstretched but don't let one hand come out in front of the other. Taking a big inhale, slowly start sliding your hands down the yardstick, dropping your head down between your arms as you're exhaling your breath. Slide your hands down the yardstick bending as far forward at your waist as possible. Your legs should be extended as far out as is comfortable for you without your knees hurting. Your score will be the most distant point in inches you reach with your fingertips on the yardstick. Do two warm-ups first and then the final test.

SOME BASIC RULES ON HOW TO STRETCH PROPERLY

Although stretching comes naturally to our bodies, there are some important instructions you should follow in order to get the most out of your stretch routine and help prevent overstretching and possible injury.

1. Never stretch cold muscles. If you like to stretch first thing in the morning, I suggest walking around your house for a few minutes to heat up your body. Another good time to stretch is after a warm bath or a shower. Again, this will raise your body temperature so you're not stretching cold muscles which could lead to an injury. If you are working out in the gym and you plan to stretch before your workout, either drive to the gym with the car heater on to warm you up, or use one of the pieces of aerobic equipment in the gym from three to five minutes first.

2. Always stretch slowly. My tango teacher always tells me dancing tango is not a race. The same is true of stretching. To get the most out of your stretches, do them slowly and with controlled movement. You often see the players on the field before a baseball game doing all these vigorous, bouncing stretches to get ready to play ball. This is called ballistic stretching. I do not recommend it for you. Slow, static stretching will help increase your flexibility and range of motion, and is safer for your body.

3. Breathe properly through the stretch. Before you move into any stretch, take a deep breath. As you lower into the stretch, exhale your breath slowly. This allows you to move into the stretch smoothly, relaxing your entire body without holding onto tension in your muscles or joints.

4. Stay in the stretch postures. Your stretches should be held for between fifteen and sixty seconds. Some stretches can be held for even longer, if they feel good and you want to pay special attention to a tight area.

5. Go deeper into a stretch. If you want to increase your stretch further while already in a stretch position, inhale deeply and as you exhale, release your body further into the stretch.

6. Enjoy the sensation. Stretching feels good. It really is an enjoyable process. Animals do it naturally because inherently they sense it is good for their bodies. In many ways, we bipedal animals have evolved away from what comes natural to our bodies and this is one of the reasons we have so many injuries related to inflexibility. While you are stretching, take a moment to appreciate how your muscles feel, visualize them stretching, monitor your breathing as you lengthen into the stretch, appreciate the fact you're doing something not only healthful for your body, but relaxing for your mind.

Body Preserving Exercises—Stretching

1 Hamstring Stretch: Single Leg Knee to Chest
2 Quadriceps Stretch: Side-Lying Bent-Leg Stretch
3 Chest and Spinal Stretch: Hyper-Arch on Exercise Ball
4 One Leg Forward Flexion
5 Piriformis Stretch
6 Spinal Twist Stretch
7 Biceps Stretch
8 Triceps Stretch

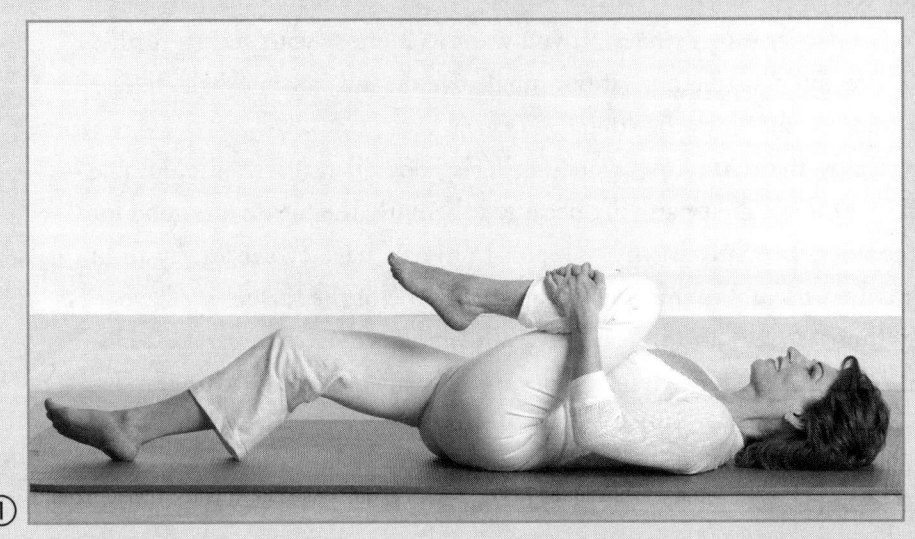

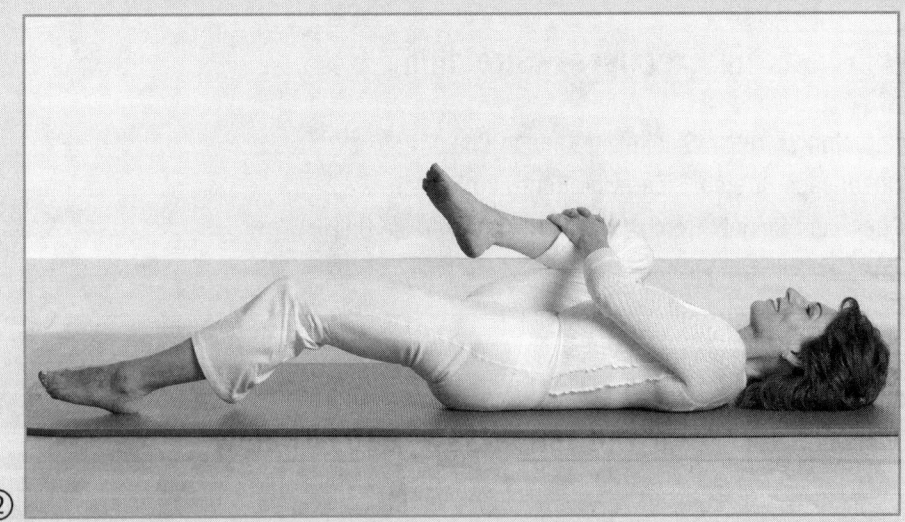

Hamstring Stretch:
Single Leg Knee to Chest

EXECUTION

Lie on your back on a firm but not hard surface. If you are doing these at home and you don't have carpet, do them on an exercise mat for comfort and to protect your spine. Bend the knee of the leg you are stretching and bring it toward your chest so you are hugging your thigh to your chest. Place both your hands below your knee, not on it, to increase the stretch. If you feel any discomfort in this position in your lower back, bring the non-working leg up so there is a slight bend at the knee.

Muscle Being Stretched:
Back of Legs—Hamstrings

Equipment:
None Required

Degree of Difficulty:
One Dumbbell

Body Position:
Supine (Lying on Back)

Form Watch:
If you feel this more in your knee than the back of your leg, place your hands behind your thigh and pull your leg toward your chest until you feel the muscles stretching in the back of your leg.

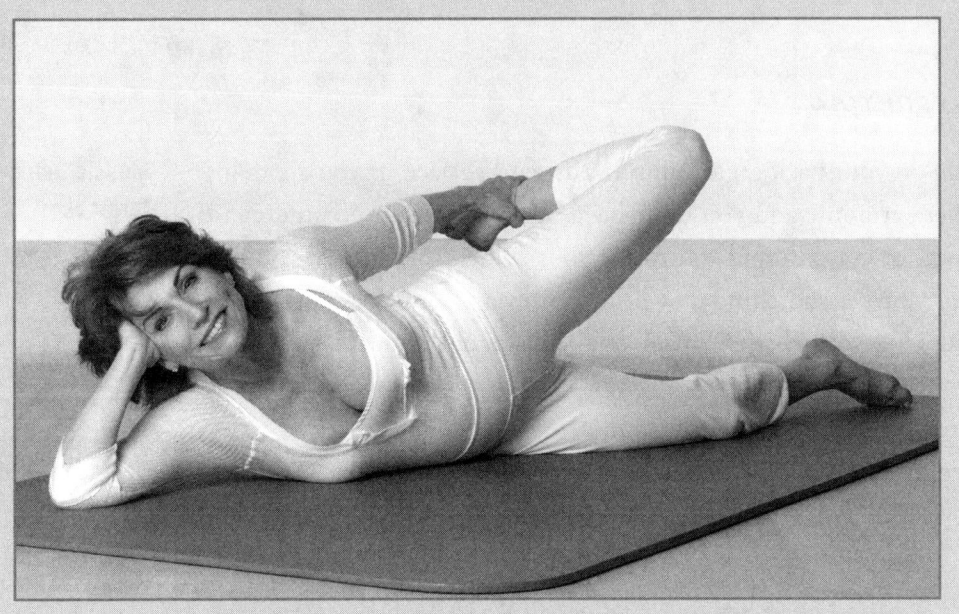

Quadriceps Stretch:
Side-Lying Bent-Leg Stretch

EXECUTION

Lie on your side so your head is resting comfortably either on your outstretched arm or in your hand. You can bend your bottom leg or keep it straight. Bend your top leg behind you so you can grab the lower part of your leg around your ankle. Gently pull your entire leg behind you until you feel a stretch in the front. If you feel this more in your knee, open up your leg so your knee is less bent and then pull your foot toward your buttocks.

Muscle Being Stretched
Front of Legs—Quadriceps

Equipment:
None Required

Degree of Difficulty:
One Dumbbell

Body Position:
Lying on Side

Form Watch:
To increase the stretch, when your leg is behind you, gently pull your foot closer to your buttocks.

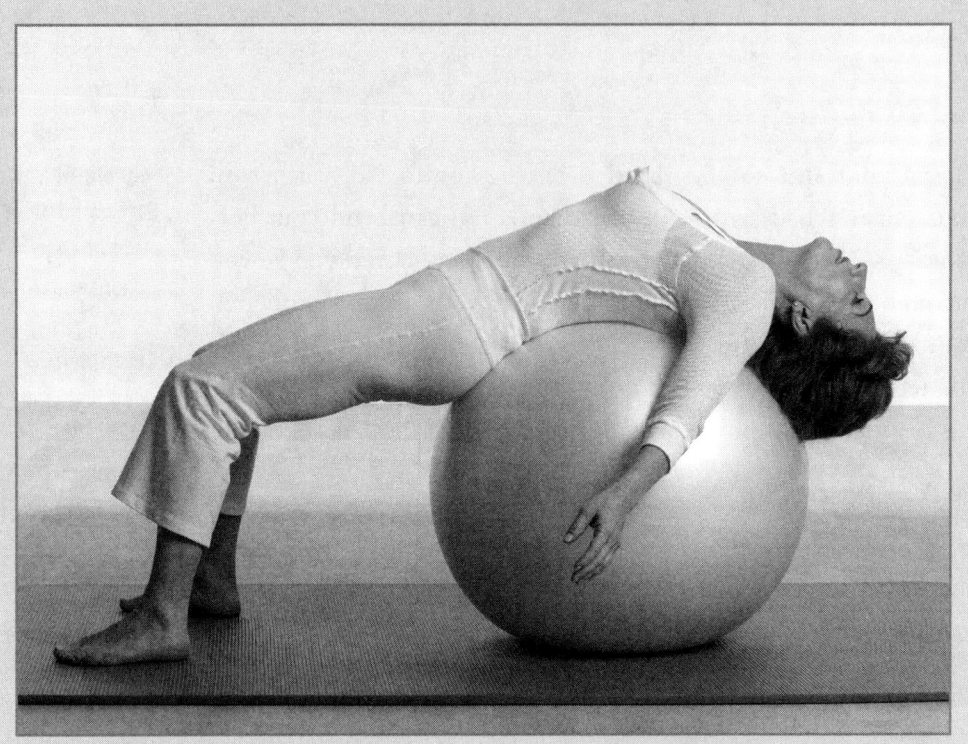

Chest and Spinal Stretch: Hyper-Arch on Exercise Ball

EXECUTION

Sit on an exercise ball and slowly roll it behind you so you can lean over and place your back comfortably over it. Place your feet away from the ball and about hip-distance apart so you feel secure on the ball. Your upper back should rest on the ball so you can allow your arms to fall to the sides. You will feel a long stretch across your chest. You will also feel an opening of the vertebrae in your back. This is a very relaxing stretch and excellent to relieve any tension in the back, shoulders, and neck.

Muscles Being Stretched:
Chest (Pectoralis) and Spine (Erector Spinae) Lower Back (Lumbar Region)

Equipment:
Exercise Ball

Degree of Difficulty:
Two Dumbbells

Body Position:
Supine (Lying on Back)

Form Watch:
Roll the ball back and forth and feel a massaging sensation on your upper and lower back.

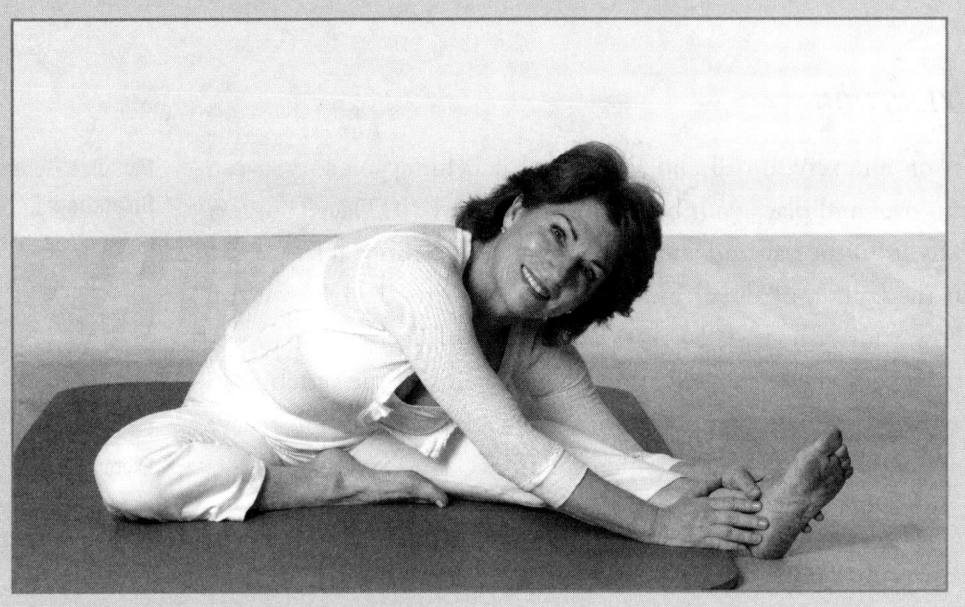

One Leg Forward Flexion

EXECUTION

Sitting on the floor, fold one leg into your body, bringing your foot in as close as possible to the thigh of your outstretched leg. Sit up tall, pulling out of your hips and bring your arms up over your head so you feel a stretch in your torso. Take a deep inhalation of air and then slowly start to release the air as you bend over at the waist, dropping your hands down to rest on your outstretched leg. Try to bring your chest as close as possible to your upper thigh, without bouncing or forcing the stretch. You will feel a stretch in the upper inner thigh and also a nice lengthening of the muscles in your lower back.

Muscles Being Stretched:
Back of Legs (Hamstrings) and Lower Back (Lumbar Region)

Equipment:
None Required

Degree of Difficulty:
One Dumbbell

Body Position:
Sitting

Form Watch:
Keep your abdominal muscles contracted and let your shoulders and neck relax in the outstretched position.

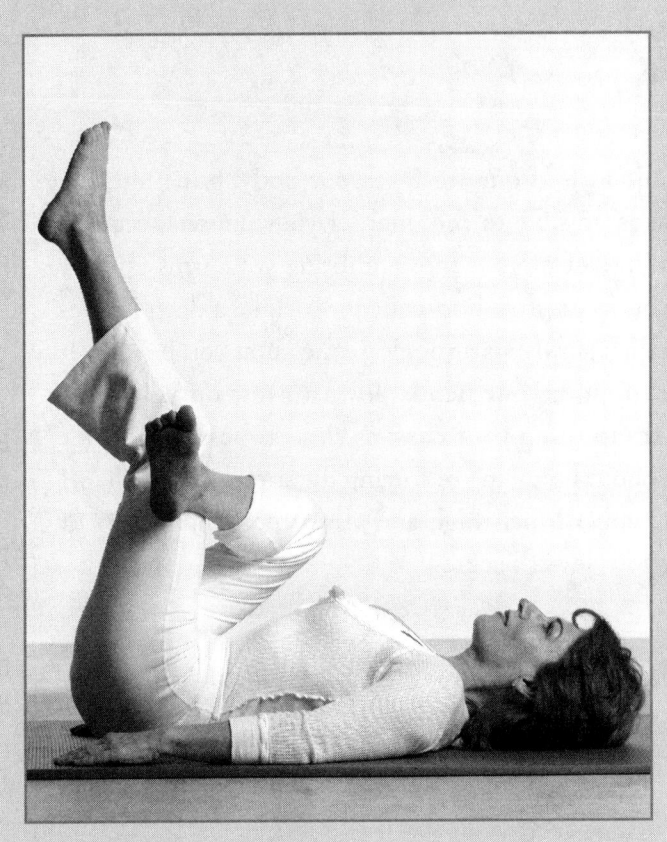

Piriformis Stretch

EXECUTION

Your piriformis muscle is one of the lateral rotator muscles located deep in your gluteal region. It is responsible for the lateral rotation of your hip. It is a muscle that frequently comes into use for those who participate in activities that require change of direction—tennis, for instance, or tango dancing.

Lying on your back on a firm, but not hard surface, cross one leg over the thigh of the other, just as you might while sitting in a chair. Lift the bottom leg up so it is straight above you while maintaining a slight bend at the knee. Use it to push the crossed leg toward your chest. Feel the stretch in your buttocks and hips.

Muscle Being Stretched:
Piriformis, Back of Legs (Hamstrings), and Lower Back (Lumbar Region)

Equipment:
None Required

Degree of Difficulty:
One Dumbbell

Body Position:
Supine (Lying on Back)

Form Watch:
To make the stretch even more intense, you can place your hands around the straight leg and pull it toward your chest even closer.

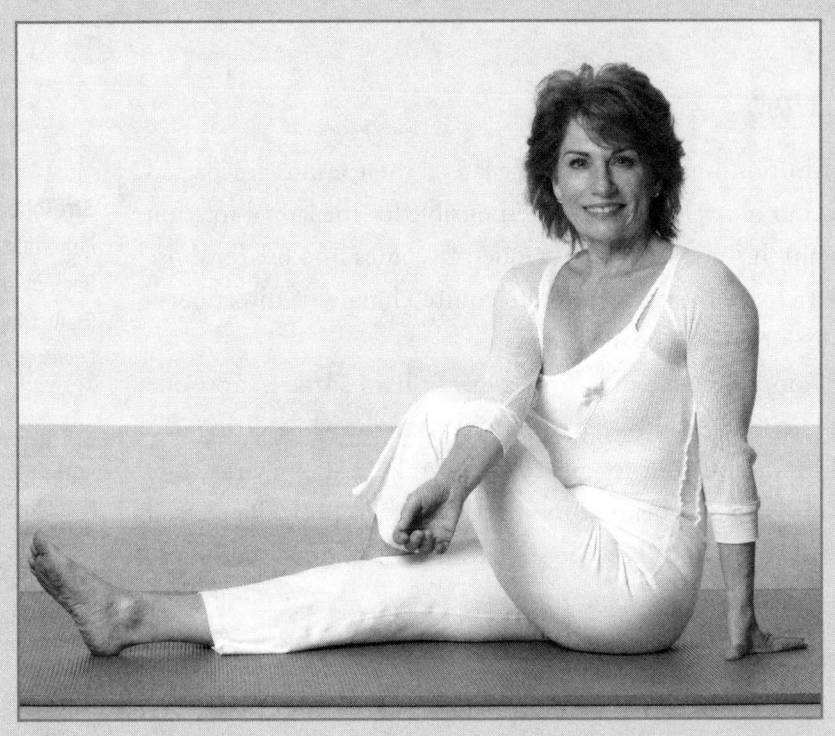

Spinal Twist Stretch

EXECUTION

Sit on the ground with good posture, contracting your abdominal muscles. Start with both legs stretched out in front of you. Take one leg and cross it over the outstretched leg so your foot is next to your thigh. Take the opposite arm from the crossed-over leg and place it on the outside of your leg, almost next to your knee. Place your other hand behind you, as close to your buttocks as possible to help you maintain a straight posture. Slowly turn your torso, using the pressure from the arm across your leg to help you execute the twist. You can repeat on the opposite side by switching arms and twisting in the opposite direction.

Muscle Being Stretched:
Lower Back (Lumbar Region)

Equipment:
None Required

Degree of Difficulty:
Two Dumbbells

Body Position:
Sitting Up

Form Watch:
Keeping your abdominals contracted will help you maintain the straight spine position essential to do this stretch correctly.

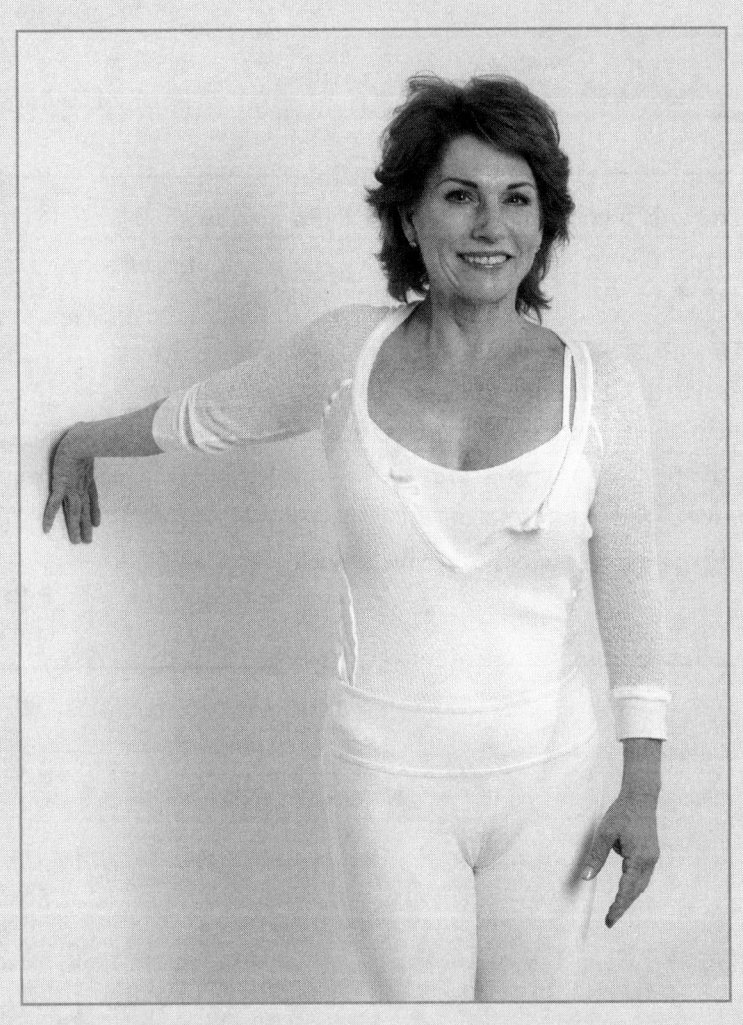

Biceps Stretch

EXECUTION

Place the hand of the arm you want to stretch against a wall, doorjam, or any object that is stationary. Your hand should be placed about two inches below the top of your shoulder. The fingertips of your hand should be turned toward the ground as much as possible and your thumb outstretched. Slowly turn your torso away from your outstretched arm until you feel a stretch in the biceps muscles.

Muscle Being Stretched:
Front of Arm—Biceps

Equipment:
None Required

Degree of Difficulty:
One Dumbbell

Body Position:
Standing

Form Watch:
If you do not feel the stretch, adjust your hand on the wall to a position allowing you to feel the stretch across the biceps.

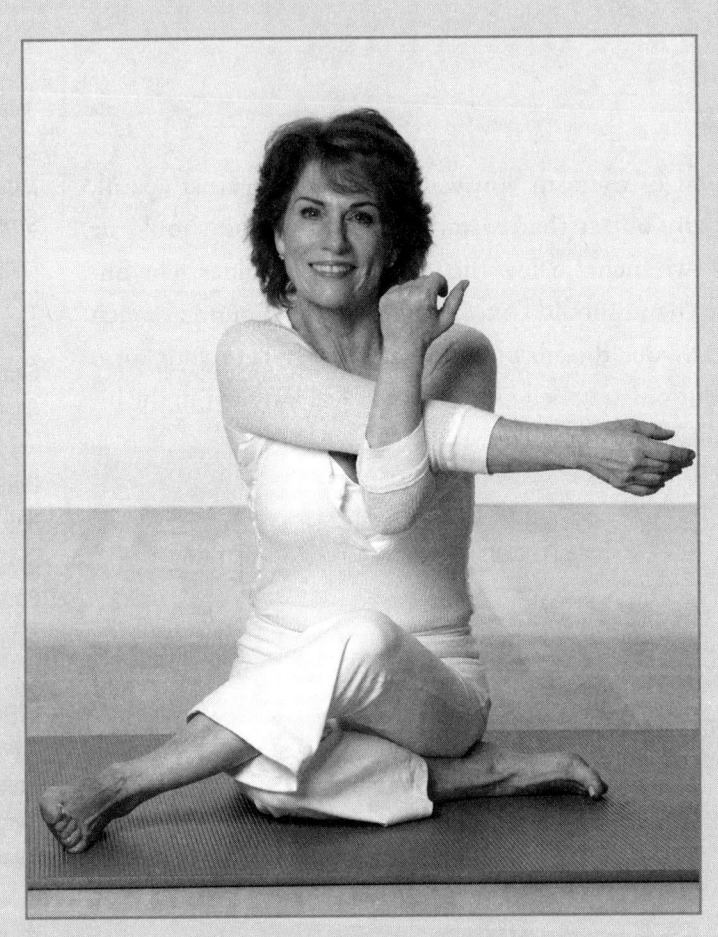

Triceps Stretch

EXECUTION

Cross the arm of the triceps muscles you are going to stretch across your body, keeping it parallel to your chest. Take your other arm and wrap it under the outstretched arm, just above the elbow. Use it to hug your outstretched arm close to your chest. You will feel a stretch in the triceps muscles.

Muscle Being Stretched:
Back of Arm—Triceps

Equipment:
None Required

Degree of Difficulty:
One Dumbbell

Body Position:
Standing or Sitting

Form Watch:
Do not rotate your body or turn at the waist, simply pull the arm to be stretched tight into the body and feel the lengthening of the triceps muscles.

The Life Balancing Exercises

Tous les jours, à tous points de vue, je vais de mieux en mieux.

ÉMILE COUÉ

"Every day, in every way, I am getting better and better," was the phrase of self inspiration coined by the renowned French psychotherapist, Émile Coué, who fostered a practice called autosuggestion. This mantra was to be uttered fifteen to twenty times a day, morning and evening.

It makes sense to recognize and acknowledge ourselves and our needs, transforming our beliefs into reality by giving them a voice.

In my first book, *Smart Girls Do Dumbbells,* I talk about the intimate connection between physical strength and personal power. I have seen this awe-inspiring transformation happen with the hundreds of women of all ages with whom I have worked over the last two decades. They start out building muscle because they want to lose weight or they have health issues and then suddenly, along the way, they start building personal power. I have seen women's lives change dramatically—ones who were once fearful and wary, take charge; some who had spent years hiding their inner beauty because of the shame they felt over their outer appearance. Women who have held themselves back suddenly blossom into forceful and fearless creatures. They start feeling they have control, not only over their bodies, but over their lives. As physical strength increases, confidence soars. It is inspirational to watch.

I created the *Life Balancing Exercises* to help coalesce your emerging physical strength with your spiritual growth and personal well-being. They are specifically designed to help you navigate the menopausal passage, which is not only a physiological transition, but for many women a profoundly emotional one as well.

LIFE BALANCING EXERCISE 1: FINDING YOUR CENTER

In Anti-Aging Exercise Strategy 9, I talk about your core, your central body strengthening. Once your core is strong, you have the stability required to experiment with all manner of movement without fear of risk of injury. The same is true of your psychological center. When we feel unbalanced, out of control, uncertain, our spirit, like our strength, flags. As with the exercises that strengthen your body's core, we each have activities, pastimes, or methods that help re-stabilize our minds and our spirits. My friend Lori's Life Centering activities include playing tennis and writing short fiction comedy stories. My friend Nancy finds solace in her art studio where she paints beautiful portraits. After a high-stress day at her work, Carole heads to the shopping mall and makes certain she doesn't miss her weekend tennis matches.

My Life Centering activities include: writing in my journal, tango dancing, watching the Red Sox play baseball, going for a walk while listening to my favorite jazz artists, having dinner with friends, and reading classical fiction.

On a sheet of paper or in a Life Balancing journal, write your Life Centering activities. Whatever those activities are for you, write them down and remember to access them on those difficult, stressful, or out-of-control days when your life is tottering on the edge.

As the Core Exercises help strengthen your body, these interventions will help bolster your spirits.

LIFE BALANCING EXERCISE 2: SELF SUPPORT

Many of us never imagine we will have to take care of ourselves. If unmarried, perhaps we are waiting for "Mr. Right" to come along before buying a house, going for an advanced degree, or traveling to Italy. If married, we've mostly relied on our spouse to make the important decisions, such as the financial decisions. When life's hard realities hit, we are totally unprepared and overwhelmed by our dependency on someone else to take care of us.

In Anti-Aging Exercise Strategy 3, I give you exercises to help you build stronger leg muscles. You need physical strength to maintain your functional mobility and freedom of movement; you need some basic financial and life-management skills to maintain your independence. For instance, do you know what benefits are available to you for financial support through the Social Security office should you become widowed or divorced? Do you even know your husband's social security number? You should. Do you know how much you owe on your home? Or, if there is an equity line on it? Do you have credit card debt? If so, what interest rate are you paying? What stocks and bonds do you own? What type of health insurance coverage do you have? There is a lot of free information for women at various financial websites. Here is the web address for Social Security: www.ssa.gov. which is a great website to answer some basic questions.

If you haven't done so before, now is the time to gather important information about your personal finances. Write down five things you have done to take care of yourself and your family financially and five things you need to do, and a timeline for accomplishing these tasks.

LIFE BALANCING EXERCISE 3:
BANKING ON YOUR ASSETS

Every woman possesses a magnificent feature, skill, talent, or trait. Whatever your unique gift is, it belongs to you. It's what sets you apart and makes you the compelling woman you are. But too often women step away from themselves, don't embrace their glory, or they downplay their accomplishments or physical assets.

I work privately with a woman who will never be slim, but she exercises with me three times a week and she's never been in better shape or health. She has the most perfectly shaped lips I have ever seen and a lovely smile.

But, she never wore lipstick, not even a little gloss to enhance her beautiful mouth. I always commented to her on her beautiful smile, but she would just shrug it off. After we'd worked together for about seven months and she'd lost about fourteen pounds and was really getting strong and fit, one day she came to workout and she was wearing this magnificent color of lipstick and she looked radiant!

When I told her she looked incredible and asked her what made her put on lipstick she said, "I feel so much better about myself these days. I think I can handle some attention now."

In Anti-Aging Exercise Strategy 4 I give you Body Preserving Exercises for building your extensor muscles—your buttocks and hips. These are the muscles that propel you into forward movement—walking, running, jogging. As the strength in our extensor muscles gain power, so should the strength in our self esteem and pride, which also move us in a forward direction toward personal power.

Write out the three physical assets of which you are most proud and three character assets that define who you are, and what it is that makes you proud of these traits or behaviors.

LIFE BALANCING EXERCISE 4: DREAM SEEKING

We all harbor some special dream or aspiration. We may even label the dream we secretly cherish as being crazy or silly. It might be doing stand-up comedy, writing a play, dancing in a tango show (that's mine), or singing in a nightclub. It might be an act of daring-do, like skydiving or high altitude mountain climbing.

But still, it is our dream. Often times the only thing preventing us from pursuing our secret desire is fear—fear of failure, of looking foolish, of being criticized, or of being *too old*.

In Anti-Aging Exercise Strategy 8 I talk about how strong shoulders give us a striking presentation in the world and how they provide structural strength to our entire upper body and carriage. The stronger we become physically, the more courage we possess to take risks and pursue our dreams.

Name a secret dream, fantasy, or aspiration and three steps you would take to turn that dream into a reality.

LIFE BALANCING EXERCISE 5: WORDS OF WISDOM

What words of wisdom inspire you, give you courage, confidence, and solace? Maybe a line from a movie, a musical, a play, or a poem. Maybe something you read in a novel or a sign you saw walking down the street. If it strengthens your soul as exercise does your body, jot it down in your Life Balancing journal, a diary, or just on a scrap of paper you keep by your bed or in your wallet.

I was recently attending a business conference in Los Angeles and I went to a panel featuring two of the world's greatest athletes, Andre Agassi and Lance Armstrong. When Agassi spoke about physical health he said, "A strong body obeys, a weak body commands." He went on to define further what he meant by explaining that when your body is weak it tells you what to do, when your body is strong, you tell it what to do. I immediately wrote these words down on a paper napkin and when I got home transferred them to my Life Balancing journal so I would remember them to share with you now.

Write down some meaningful words, an expression or thoughts that you recall gave you a sense of comfort, made you laugh, or had a special meaning. It doesn't have to be the exact wording, just the essence of the meaning. And then add to this collection. Whenever you hear or read or see something that strikes you as meaningful, write it down. You will soon possess your own compendium of inspirational wisdom.

SECTION TWO

THE 6-WEEK BODY & HEALTH RECLAMATION PROGRAMS

INTRODUCTION TO THE SYSTEMS

ANTI-AGING WORKOUT SYSTEM 1
Goal: Weight Loss, Tone, and Firm

ANTI-AGING WORKOUT SYSTEM 2
Goal: Increase Strength, Tone, and Firm

ANTI-AGING WORKOUT SYSTEM 3
Goal: Cardiovascular Health, Tone, and Firm

MASTER ANTI-AGING EXERCISE GRID

Introduction to
the Systems

THE ANTI-AGING WORKOUT SYSTEMS

- Goal: Weight Loss, Tone, and Firm
- Goal: Increase Strength, Tone, and Firm
- Goal: Cardiovascular Health, Tone, and Firm

The three Anti-Aging Workout Systems that follow are 6-Week, Day-by-Day customized programs designed specifically to help you achieve and maintain your personal health and fitness goals.

Each Anti-Aging Workout System is a complete program itself, but they are also totally modular in design so that you can move from one system to another without losing any of your workout days or results.

One of the biggest complaints I hear from my clients and from my patients while at UCLA is, "exercise is boring." It is one of the leading culprits why people stop working out. And that makes perfectly good sense. If every time you worked out you did the exact same program, day in and day out, of course you'd become bored and disenchanted. Just like anything else you do over and over and over again without changing it up or adding variety, eventually you'd come to the not inaccurate conclusion: "this is so boring, I can't do it

[211]

anymore." (I've been at the place myself.) And even if you could force yourself to do it, your enthusiasm and commitment would be severely compromised and eventually you probably wouldn't be getting the results you desired.

The Muscle Your Way Through Menopause...and Beyond Anti-Aging Workout Systems eliminate the "boredom" factor because each day you are doing a new workout program. They are also designed so you can complete some of the programs in around thirty minutes, and none should take you any longer than fifty minutes.

When you complete your first 6-Week Anti-Aging Workout System, you then have the option to continue to follow it as is, to change it around, or inter-mix it with any of the other Workout Systems. The ultimate goal is for you to find a program that best suits your needs, allowing you to achieve the health and fitness results you desire, and most importantly, one that you enjoy doing and can remain with...forever!

SOME IMPORTANT PROGRAMMING NOTES
EVALUATING YOUR FITNESS LEVEL

Beginner:

You would follow the sets and reps for a beginner if you:

- Have never participated in any formal exercise program.
- Haven't done any exercise in over twenty-four months.
- Never used weight training equipment—dumbbells, barbells, exercise machines.
- Feel uncertain about how to do any of the exercises.

Intermediate:

You would follow the sets and reps for an intermediate exerciser if you:

- Have been regularly participating in an exercise program from two to three days a week for the last twelve months.
- Have some knowledge and understanding of how to properly use weight training equipment.
- Desire to achieve greater results and are ready to increase your workout program.

Advanced:

You would follow the sets and reps for an advanced exerciser if you:

- Have been exercising regularly at least three days a week or more for at least twelve months.
- Feel comfortable using weight equipment.
- Feel you are doing your exercises with proper form and technique.
- Enjoy the process of exercising and have a desire to work at an advanced level.

SELECTING THE APPROPRIATE SIZE WEIGHTS

You can never go wrong by selecting a low weight to start. This is especially true if you are a beginner or if an exercise is new to you. As you gain strength, you will slowly move up to the next size weights. Increase the size of the weights you are using when:

- You can do the last three reps of your last set easily without sacrificing your form and technique.
- You want to be more challenged.
- You've been using the same size weights for over six months and you want to achieve greater results.

Consult with Your Physician

Prior to beginning or changing any exercise program, consult with your physician. If you have any questions about what Anti-Aging Workout System is the best for you, bring *Muscle Your Way Through Menopause . . . and Beyond* to your doctor and go over the various options together.

I've given you more than 80 exercise options and 126 daily exercise programs. If an exercise does not feel right to you, if you don't like it or if it is too difficult, don't do it! Choose exercises that you feel you can do correctly, consistently, and will help you achieve your health and fitness goals.

In my book, *Smart Girls Do Dumbbells*, I include a chapter called "You Are Your Own Best Coach." What I mean by this is you know your own body better than anyone else. Trust your instincts. Never do any exercise that is too difficult for your skill level, doesn't feel right for your body, or you just don't like.

If you have any questions regarding any of the Anti-Aging Exercise Strategies or the Anti-Aging Workout Systems, feel free to email me at: judith@smartgirlsdodumbbells.com.

ANTI-AGING WORKOUT SYSTEM 1
Goal: Weight Loss, Tone, and Firm

WEIGHT LOSS: WEEK ONE/ DAY 1

Aerobic

EXERCISE OPTIONS:	TIME:
Walking/Treadmill/Swimming/Biking/ Elliptical, Stairmaster/Aerobic Video	20 Minutes Heart Rate Goal: Between 65%–75%

Core

EXERCISE	FITNESS LEVEL	SETS	REPS
Classic Crunches	Beginner	1	8–10
	Intermediate	2	10–12
	Advanced	3	10–15
Cycle Rotations	Beginner	1	8–10
	Intermediate	2	10–12
	Advanced	3	12–15
Reverse Leg Lifts Using Ankle Weights	Beginner	1	8–10
	Intermediate	2	10–12
	Advanced	3	10–15

Stretch

EXERCISE	SETS	HOLD
Hamstring Stretch: Single Leg Knee to Chest	3	15–60 Seconds
Piriformis Stretch	3	15–60 Seconds
Spinal Twist	3	15–60 Seconds

WEIGHT LOSS: WEEK ONE/ DAY 2

Aerobic

EXERCISE OPTIONS:	TIME:
Walking/Treadmill/Swimming/Biking/ Elliptical, Stairmaster/Aerobic	10 Minutes Heart Rate Goal: Between 65%–75%

Strength Training: Upper Body

CHOOSE ONE EXERCISE FOR EACH BODY PART:

SETS AND REPS:

Beginner:
Sets: 1
Reps: 8–10

Intermediate:
Sets: 2
Reps: 10–12

Advanced:
Sets: 3
Reps: 12–15

Chest
- Ball Push-Ups
- Chest Press on Bench Using Body Bar or Smith Machine
- Dumbbell Presses Over Exercise Ball
- Wall Push-Ups*

Back
- Lat Pull-Downs
- One-Arm Kneeling Rows
- Machine Assisted Pull-Ups
- Back Rows*

Biceps
- Biceps Curls Using Dumbbells
- Body Bar Biceps Curls
- Cable Biceps Curls
- Isometric Biceps Curls*

Triceps
- Triceps Extensions Pull-Downs
- One-Arm Overhead Triceps Extension
- Lying Triceps Extension
- Triceps V-Backs*

Shoulders
- Side Arm Raises Using Dumbbells
- Overhead Presses Using Dumbbells
- Reverse Flyes on Ball Using Dumbbells
- Reverse Flyes*

*Equipment-Free Exercises

Core

EXERCISE	FITNESS LEVEL	SETS	REPS
Ball Crunches	Beginner	1	8–10
	Intermediate	2	10–12
	Advanced	3	10–15
Lateral Side Drops on Ball	Beginner	1	8–10
	Intermediate	2	10–12
	Advanced	3	12–15
Sitting Leg Lifts	Beginner	1	8–10
	Intermediate	2	10–12
	Advanced	3	10–15

Stretch

EXERCISE	SETS	HOLD
Hamstring Stretch: Single Leg Knee to Chest	3	15–60 Seconds
Piriformis Stretch	3	15–60 Seconds
Biceps/Triceps Stretches	3	15–60 Seconds

WEIGHT LOSS: WEEK ONE/ DAY 3

Aerobic

EXERCISE OPTIONS:	TIME:
Walking/Treadmill/Swimming/Biking/ Elliptical, Stairmaster/Aerobic Video	20 Minutes Heart Rate Goal: Between 65%–75%

Core

EXERCISE	FITNESS LEVEL	SETS	REPS
Reverse Leg Lifts with Ankle Weights	Beginner	1	8–10
	Intermediate	2	10–12
	Advanced	3	10–15
Cycle Rotations	Beginner	1	8–10
	Intermediate	2	10–12
	Advanced	3	12–15
Back Extensions on Exercise Ball	Beginner	1	8–10
	Intermediate	2	10–12
	Advanced	3	10–15

Stretch

EXERCISE	SETS	HOLD
One Leg Forward Flexion	3	15–60 Seconds
Hyper-Arch on Exercise Ball	3	15–60 Seconds
Spinal Twist	3	15–60 Seconds

WEIGHT LOSS: WEEK ONE/ DAY 4

Aerobic

EXERCISE OPTIONS:	TIME:
Walking/Treadmill/Swimming/Biking/ Elliptical, Stairmaster/Aerobic	10 Minutes Heart Rate Goal: Between 65%–75%

―――――――― *Strength Training: Lower Body* ――――――――

CHOOSE ONE EXERCISE FOR EACH BODY PART:

SETS AND REPS:

Beginner:
Sets: 1
Reps: 8–10

Intermediate:
Sets: 2
Reps: 10–12

Advanced:
Sets: 3
Reps: 12–15

Glutes and Hips
- Ball Squats
- Side-Lying Leg Lifts Using Exercise Band
- Reverse Lunges Using Ankle Weights
- Sit Downs*

Front of Legs
- Plié Squats Against Ball
- Seated Leg Extension
- Leg Extensions Using Ankle Weights
- Lying Bent Knee Leg Lifts*

Back of Legs
- Standing Hamstring Curls Using Ankle Weights

- Hamstring Curls Using Ankle Weights Over Bench, Chair or Ball
- Machine Hamstring Curls
- Standing Hamstring Curls*

Calves
- Standing Heel Raises Using Dumbbells
- Machine Heel Raises
- Heel Raises*

*Equipment-Free Exercise

―――――――――――――――― *Core* ――――――――――――――――

EXERCISE	FITNESS LEVEL	SETS	REPS
Plank or Modified Plank	Beginner	1	8–10
	Intermediate	2	10–12
	Advanced	3	10–15
Ball Crunches	Beginner	1	8–10
	Intermediate	2	10–12
	Advanced	3	12–15
Kegels	Beginner	1	8–10
	Intermediate	2	10–12
	Advanced	3	10–15

―――――――――――――――― *Stretch* ――――――――――――――――

EXERCISE	SETS	HOLD
Hamstring Stretch: Single Leg Knee to Chest	3	15–60 Seconds
Quadriceps Stretch: Side-Lying Bent-Leg Stretch	3	15–60 Seconds
Hyper-Arch on Exercise Ball	3	15–60 Seconds

WEIGHT LOSS: WEEK ONE/ DAY 5

Aerobic

EXERCISE OPTIONS:	TIME:
Walking/Treadmill/Swimming/Biking/ Elliptical, Stairmaster/Aerobic Video	20 Minutes Heart Rate Goal: Between 65%–75%

Core

EXERCISE	FITNESS LEVEL	SETS	REPS
Isometric Squeezes	Beginner	1	8–10
	Intermediate	2	10–12
	Advanced	3	10–15
Pelvic Tilts	Beginner	1	8–10
	Intermediate	2	10–12
	Advanced	3	12–15
Crunches on Flat Bench Using Resistance Ball	Beginner	1	8–10
	Intermediate	2	10–12
	Advanced	3	10–15

Stretch

EXERCISE	SETS	HOLD
Spinal Twist	3	15–60 Seconds
Hyper-Arch on Exercise Ball	3	15–60 Seconds
Piriformis Stretch	3	15–60 Seconds

WEIGHT LOSS: WEEK ONE/ DAY 6

Aerobic

EXERCISE OPTIONS:	TIME:
Walking/Treadmill/Swimming/Biking/ Elliptical, Stairmaster/Aerobic	10 Minutes Heart Rate Goal: Between 65%–75%

——————————— *Strength Training: Upper Body* ———————————

CHOOSE ONE EXERCISE FOR EACH BODY PART:

SETS AND REPS:

Beginner:
Sets: 1
Reps: 8–10

Intermediate:
Sets: 2
Reps: 10–12

Advanced:
Sets: 3
Reps: 12–15

Chest
- Chest Flyes Using Dumbbells on Flat Bench
- Chest Press on Bench Using Body Bar or Smith Machine
- Dumbbell Presses Over Exercise Ball
- Floor Push-Ups*

Back
- Lat Pull-Downs
- One-Arm Kneeling Rows
- Bent-Over Body Bar Rows
- Arm Pull-Downs*

Biceps
- Biceps Curls Using Dumbbells

- Seated One-Arm Biceps Curls
- Cable Biceps Curls
- Isometric Biceps Curls*

Triceps
- Triceps Extension Pull-Downs
- One-Arm Overhead Triceps Extension
- Lying Triceps Extension
- Triceps Wall Push-Ups*

Shoulders
- Angled One-Arm Side Raises
- Overhead Presses Using Dumbbells
- Reverse Flyes on Ball Using Dumbbells
- Reverse Flyes*

*Equipment-Free Exercises

——————————— *Core* ———————————

EXERCISE	FITNESS LEVEL	SETS	REPS
Back Extensions on Exercise Ball	Beginner	1	8–10
	Intermediate	2	10–12
	Advanced	3	10–15
Cycle Rotations	Beginner	1	8–10
	Intermediate	2	10–12
	Advanced	3	12–15
Sitting Leg Lifts	Beginner	1	8–10
	Intermediate	2	10–12
	Advanced	3	10–15

——————————— *Stretch* ———————————

EXERCISE	SETS	HOLD
One Leg Forward Flexion	3	15–60 Seconds
Piriformis Stretch	3	15–60 Seconds
Spinal Twist	3	15–60 Seconds

WEIGHT LOSS: WEEK ONE/ DAY 7
OPTIONAL: REST DAY

Aerobic

EXERCISE OPTIONS:	TIME:
Walking/Treadmill/Swimming/Biking/ Elliptical, Stairmaster/Aerobic Video	15 Minutes Heart Rate Goal: Between 65%–75%

Core

EXERCISE	FITNESS LEVEL	SETS	REPS
Leg Lifts	Beginner	1	8–10
	Intermediate	2	10–12
	Advanced	3	10–15
Kegels	Beginner	1	8–10
	Intermediate	2	10–12
	Advanced	3	12–15
Pelvic Tilts	Beginner	1	8–10
	Intermediate	2	10–12
	Advanced	3	10–15

Stretch

EXERCISE	SETS	HOLD
Hamstring Stretch: Single Leg Knee to Chest	3	15–60 Seconds
Hyper-Arch on Exercise Ball	3	15–60 Seconds
One Leg Forward Flexion	3	15–60 Seconds

WEIGHT LOSS: WEEK TWO/ DAY 1

Aerobic

EXERCISE OPTIONS:	TIME:
Walking/Treadmill/Swimming/Biking/ Elliptical, Stairmaster/Aerobic Video	25 Minutes Heart Rate Goal: Between 65%–75%

Core

EXERCISE	FITNESS LEVEL	SETS	REPS
Ball Crunches	Beginner	1	8–10
	Intermediate	2	10–12
	Advanced	3	10–15
Lateral Side Drops on Ball	Beginner	1	8–10
	Intermediate	2	10–12
	Advanced	3	12–15
Reverse Leg Lifts with Ankle Weights	Beginner	1	8–10
	Intermediate	2	10–12
	Advanced	3	10–15

Stretch

EXERCISE	SETS	HOLD
Hamstring Stretch: Single Leg Knee to Chest	3	15–60 Seconds
Piriformis Stretch	3	15–60 Seconds
Spinal Twist	3	15–60 Seconds

WEIGHT LOSS: WEEK TWO/ DAY 2

Aerobic

EXERCISE OPTIONS:	TIME:
Walking/Treadmill/Swimming/Biking/ Elliptical, Stairmaster/Aerobic	10 Minutes Heart Rate Goal: Between 65%–75%

--- *Strength Training: Lower Body* ---

CHOOSE ONE EXERCISE FOR EACH BODY PART:

SETS AND REPS:

Beginner:
Sets: 1
Reps: 8–10

Intermediate:
Sets: 2
Reps: 10–12

Advanced:
Sets: 3
Reps 12–15

Glutes and Hips
- Ball Squats
- Step-Ups Using Barbell or Dumbbells
- Squats on Smith Machine
- Reverse Lunges*

Front of Legs
- Leg Extensions Using Ankle Weights
- Seated Leg Extension
- Side-Lying Inner Thigh Lifts Using Ankle Weights
- Lying Bent Knee Leg Lifts*

Back of Legs
- Standing Hamstring Curls Using Ankle Weights

- Hamstring Curls Using Ankle Weights Over Bench, Chair or Ball
- Machine Hamstring Curls
- Standing Hamstring Curls*

Calves
- Standing Heel Raises Using Dumbbells
- Machine Heel Raises
- Heel Raises*

*Equipment-Free Exercises

--- Core ---

EXERCISE	FITNESS LEVEL	SETS	REPS
Leg Lifts	Beginner	1	8–10
	Intermediate	2	10–12
	Advanced	3	10–15
Crunches on Exercise Bench Using Resistance Ball	Beginner	1	8–10
	Intermediate	2	10–12
	Advanced	3	12–15
Pelvic Tilts	Beginner	1	8–10
	Intermediate	2	10–12
	Advanced	3	10–15

--- Stretch ---

EXERCISE	SETS	HOLD
One Leg Forward Flexion	3	15–60 Seconds
Quadriceps Stretch: Side-Lying Bent-Leg Stretch	3	15–60 Seconds
Hyper-Arch on Exercise Ball	3	15–60 Seconds

WEIGHT LOSS: WEEK TWO/ DAY 3

Aerobic

EXERCISE OPTIONS:	TIME:
Walking/Treadmill/Swimming/Biking/ Elliptical, Stairmaster/Aerobic Video	25 Minutes Heart Rate Goal: Between 65%–75%

Core

EXERCISE	FITNESS LEVEL	SETS	REPS
Reverse Leg Lifts Using Ankle Weights	Beginner	1	8–10
	Intermediate	2	10–12
	Advanced	3	10–15
Plank or Modified Plank	Beginner	1	8–10
	Intermediate	2	10–12
	Advanced	3	12–15
Lateral Drops on Exercise Ball	Beginner	1	8–10
	Intermediate	2	10–12
	Advanced	3	10–15

Stretch

EXERCISE	SETS	HOLD
One Leg Forward Flexion	3	15–60 Seconds
Piriformis Stretch	3	15–60 Seconds
Spinal Twist	3	15–60 Seconds

WEIGHT LOSS: WEEK TWO/ DAY 4

Aerobic

EXERCISE OPTIONS:	TIME:
Walking/Treadmill/Swimming/Biking/ Elliptical, Stairmaster/Aerobic	10 Minutes Heart Rate Goal: Between 65%–75%

Strength Training: Upper Body

CHOOSE ONE EXERCISE FOR EACH BODY PART:

SETS AND REPS:

Beginner:
Sets: 1
Reps: 8–10

Intermediate:
Sets: 2
Reps: 10–12

Advanced:
Sets: 3
Reps 12–15

Chest
- Flyes on Pec Machine
- Chest Press on Bench Using Body Bar or Smith Machine
- Dumbbell Presses Over Exercise Ball
- Presses*

Back
- Lat Pull-Downs
- Seated Low Rows
- Bent-Over Body Bar Rows
- Arm Pull-Downs

Biceps
- Biceps Curls Using Dumbbells
- Body Bar Biceps Curls
- Cable Biceps Curls
- Isometric Biceps Curls*

Triceps
- Triceps Extensions Pull-Downs
- One-Arm Overhead Triceps Extension
- Lying Triceps Extension
- Overhead Triceps Extension*

Shoulders
- One Arm Front Delt Lifts Using Dumbbells
- Shoulder Press Machine
- Reverse Flyes on Ball Using Dumbbells
- Overhead Presses

*Equipment-Free Exercises

Core

EXERCISE	FITNESS LEVEL	SETS	REPS
Classic Crunches*	Beginner	1	8–10
	Intermediate	2	10–12
	Advanced	3	10–15
Cycle Rotations	Beginner	1	8–10
	Intermediate	2	10–12
	Advanced	3	12–15
Quadruped Using Ankle Weights	Beginner	1	8–10
	Intermediate	2	10–12
	Advanced	3	10–15

Stretch

EXERCISE	SETS	HOLD
Hamstring Stretch: Single Leg Knee to Chest	3	15–60 Seconds
Hyper-Arch on Exercise Ball	3	15–60 Seconds
Biceps/Triceps Stretches	3	15–60 Seconds

WEIGHT LOSS: WEEK TWO/ DAY 5

— Aerobic —

EXERCISE OPTIONS:	TIME:
Walking/Treadmill/Swimming/Biking/ Elliptical, Stairmaster/Aerobic Video	25 Minutes Heart Rate Goal: Between 65%–75%

— Core —

EXERCISE	FITNESS LEVEL	SETS	REPS
Back Extensions on Exercise Ball	Beginner	1	8–10
	Intermediate	2	10–12
	Advanced	3	10–15
Kegels	Beginner	1	8–10
	Intermediate	2	10–12
	Advanced	3	12–15
Ball Crunches	Beginner	1	8–10
	Intermediate	2	10–12
	Advanced	3	10–15

— Stretch —

EXERCISE	SETS	HOLD
Spinal Twist	3	15–60 Seconds
Hyper-Arch on Exercise Ball	3	15–60 Seconds
Piriformis Stretch	3	15–60 Seconds

WEIGHT LOSS: WEEK TWO/ DAY 6

— Aerobic —

EXERCISE OPTIONS:	TIME:
Walking/Treadmill/Swimming/Biking/ Elliptical, Stairmaster/Aerobic	10 Minutes Heart Rate Goal: Between 65%–75%

Strength Training: Lower Body

CHOOSE ONE EXERCISE FOR EACH BODY PART

SETS AND REPS:

Beginner:
Sets: 1
Reps: 8–10

Intermediate:
Sets: 2
Reps: 10–12

Advanced:
Sets: 3
Reps 12–15

Glutes and Hips
- Side-Lying Leg Lifts Using Exercise Band
- Step-Ups Using Barbell or Dumbbells
- Single Leg Lunges Using Resistance Ball
- Stationary Lunges*

Front of Legs
- Leg Extensions Using Ankle Weights
- Seated Leg Extension
- Inner Thigh Ball Squeezes
- Lying Bent Knee Leg Lifts*

Back of Legs
- Standing Hamstring Curls Using Ankle Weights

- Hamstring Curls Using Ankle Weights Over Bench, Chair or Ball
- Machine Hamstring Curls
- Standing Hamstring Curls*

Calves
- Standing Heel Raises Using Dumbbells
- Machine Heel Raises
- Heel Raises*

*Equipment-Free Exercise

Core

EXERCISE	FITNESS LEVEL	SETS	REPS
Quadruped Using Ankle Weights	Beginner	1	8–10
	Intermediate	2	10–12
	Advanced	3	10–15
Crunches on Exercise Bench Using Resistance Ball	Beginner	1	8–10
	Intermediate	2	10–12
	Advanced	3	12–15
Pelvic Tilts	Beginner	1	8–10
	Intermediate	2	10–12
	Advanced	3	10–15

Stretch

EXERCISE	SETS	HOLD
One-Leg Forward Flexion	3	15–60 Seconds
Quadriceps Stretch: Side-Lying Bent-Leg Stretch	3	15–60 Seconds
Hyper-Arch on Exercise Ball	3	15–60 Seconds

WEIGHT LOSS: WEEK TWO/ DAY 7
OPTIONAL: REST DAY

Aerobic

EXERCISE OPTIONS:	TIME:
Walking/Treadmill/Swimming/Biking/ Elliptical, Stairmaster/Aerobic Video	15 Minutes Heart Rate Goal: Between 65%–75%

Core

EXERCISE	FITNESS LEVEL	SETS	REPS
Isometric Squeezes	Beginner	1	8–10
	Intermediate	2	10–12
	Advanced	3	10–15
Kegels	Beginner	1	8–10
	Intermediate	2	10–12
	Advanced	3	12–15
Plank or Modified Plank	Beginner	1	8–10
	Intermediate	2	10–12
	Advanced	3	10–15

Stretch

EXERCISE	SETS	HOLD
Hamstring Stretch: Single Leg Knee to Chest	3	15–60 Seconds
Spinal Twist	3	15–60 Seconds
Piriformis Stretch	3	15–60 Seconds

WEIGHT LOSS: WEEK THREE/ DAY 1

Aerobic

EXERCISE OPTIONS:	TIME:
Walking/Treadmill/Swimming/Biking/ Elliptical, Stairmaster/Aerobic Video	30 Minutes Heart Rate Goal: Between 65%–75%

Core

EXERCISE	FITNESS LEVEL	SETS	REPS
Classic Crunches*	Beginner	1	8–10
	Intermediate	2	10–12
	Advanced	3	10–15
Cycle Rotations*	Beginner	1	8–10
	Intermediate	2	10–12
	Advanced	3	12–15
Reverse Leg Lifts Using Ankle Weights	Beginner	1	8–10
	Intermediate	2	10–12
	Advanced	3	10–15

Stretch

EXERCISE	SETS	HOLD
One Leg Forward Flexion	3	15–60 Seconds
Piriformis Stretch	3	15–60 Seconds
Spinal Twist	3	15–60 Seconds

WEIGHT LOSS: WEEK THREE/ DAY 2

Aerobic

EXERCISE OPTIONS:	TIME:
Walking/Treadmill/Swimming/Biking/ Elliptical, Stairmaster/Aerobic	15 Minutes Heart Rate Goal: Between 65%–75%

Strength Training: Upper Body

CHOOSE ONE EXERCISE FOR EACH BODY PART:

SETS AND REPS:

Beginner:
Sets: 1
Reps: 8–10

Intermediate:
Sets: 2
Reps: 10–12

Advanced:
Sets: 3
Reps 12–15

Chest
- Ball Push-Ups
- Chest Press Using Body Bar/Smith Machine
- Dumbbell Presses on Ball
- Wall Push-Ups*

Back
- Lat Pull Downs
- One-Arm Kneeling Rows
- Machine Assisted Pull-Ups
- Back Rows*

Biceps
- Biceps Curls Using Dumbbells
- Body Bar Biceps Curls
- Cable Biceps Curls
- Isometric Biceps Curls*

Triceps
- Triceps Extension Pull-Downs
- One-Arm Overhead Triceps Extension
- Lying Triceps Extension
- Triceps V-Backs*

Shoulders
- One Arm Front Delt Lifts Using Dumbbells
- Shoulder Press Machine
- Reverse Flyes on Ball Using Dumbbells
- Overhead Presses*

*Equipment-Free Exercises

Core

EXERCISE	FITNESS LEVEL	SETS	REPS
Ball Crunches	Beginner	1	8–10
	Intermediate	2	10–12
	Advanced	3	10–15
Lateral Side Drops on Ball	Beginner	1	8–10
	Intermediate	2	10–12
	Advanced	3	12–15
Sitting Leg Lifts	Beginner	1	8–10
	Intermediate	2	10–12
	Advanced	3	10–15

Stretch

EXERCISE	SETS	HOLD
Hamstring Stretch: Single Leg Knee to Chest	3	15–60 Seconds
Piriformis Stretch	3	15–60 Seconds
Biceps/Triceps Stretches	3	15–60 Seconds

WEIGHT LOSS: WEEK THREE/ DAY 3

Aerobic

EXERCISE OPTIONS:	TIME:
Walking/Treadmill/Swimming/Biking/ Elliptical, Stairmaster/Aerobic Video	30 Minutes Heart Rate Goal: Between 65%–75%

Core

EXERCISE	FITNESS LEVEL	SETS	REPS
Reverse Leg Lifts with Ankle Weights	Beginner	1	8–10
	Intermediate	2	10–12
	Advanced	3	10–15
Cycle Rotations	Beginner	1	8–10
	Intermediate	2	10–12
	Advanced	3	12–15
Back Extensions on Exercise Ball	Beginner	1	8–10
	Intermediate	2	10–12
	Advanced	3	10–15

Stretch

EXERCISE	SETS	HOLD
One Leg Forward Flexion	3	15–60 Seconds
Hyper-Arch on Exercise Ball	3	15–60 Seconds
Spinal Twist	3	15–60 Seconds

WEIGHT LOSS: WEEK THREE/ DAY 4

Aerobic

EXERCISE OPTIONS:	TIME:
Walking/Treadmill/Swimming/Biking/ Elliptical, Stairmaster/Aerobic	15 Minutes Heart Rate Goal: Between 65%–75%

Strength Training: Lower Body

CHOOSE ONE EXERCISE FOR EACH BODY PART

SETS AND REPS:

Beginner:
Sets: 1
Reps: 8–10

Intermediate:
Sets: 2
Reps: 10–12

Advanced:
Sets: 3
Reps 12–15

Glutes and Hips
- Ball Squats
- Side-Lying Leg Lifts Using Exercise Band
- Reverse Lunges Using Ankle Weights
- Sit Downs*

Front of Legs
- Plié Squats Against Ball
- Seated Leg Extension
- Leg Extensions Using Ankle Weights
- Lying Bent Knee Leg Lifts*

Back of Legs
- Standing Hamstring Curls Using Ankle Weights

- Hamstring Curls Using Ankle Weights Over Bench, Chair or Ball
- Machine Hamstring Curls
- Standing Hamstring Curls*

Calves
- Standing Heel Raises Using Dumbbells
- Machine Heel Raises
- Heel Raises*

*Equipment-Free Exercise

Core

EXERCISE	FITNESS LEVEL	SETS	REPS
Plank or Modified Plank	Beginner	1	8–10
	Intermediate	2	10–12
	Advanced	3	10–15
Ball Crunches	Beginner	1	8–10
	Intermediate	2	10–12
	Advanced	3	12–15
Kegels	Beginner	1	8–10
	Intermediate	2	10–12
	Advanced	3	10–15

Stretch

EXERCISE	SETS	HOLD
Hamstring Stretch: Single Leg Knee to Chest	3	15–60 Seconds
Quadriceps Stretch: Side-Lying Bent-Leg Stretch	3	15–60 Seconds
Hyper-Arch on Exercise Ball	3	15–60 Seconds

WEIGHT LOSS: WEEK THREE/ DAY 5

Aerobic

EXERCISE OPTIONS:	TIME:
Walking/Treadmill/Swimming/Biking/ Elliptical, Stairmaster/Aerobic Video	30 Minutes Heart Rate Goal: Between 65%–75%

Core

EXERCISE	FITNESS LEVEL	SETS	REPS
Isometric Squeezes	Beginner	1	8–10
	Intermediate	2	10–12
	Advanced	3	10–15
Pelvic Tilts	Beginner	1	8–10
	Intermediate	2	10–12
	Advanced	3	12–15
Crunches on Flat Bench Using Resistance Ball	Beginner	1	8–10
	Intermediate	2	10–12
	Advanced	3	10–15

Stretch

EXERCISE	SETS	HOLD
Spinal Twist	3	15–60 Seconds
One Leg Forward Flexion	3	15–60 Seconds
Hyper-Arch on Exercise Ball	3	15–60 Seconds

WEIGHT LOSS: WEEK THREE/ DAY 6

Aerobic

EXERCISE OPTIONS:	TIME:
Walking/Treadmill/Swimming/Biking/ Elliptical, Stairmaster/Aerobic	15 Minutes Heart Rate Goal: Between 65%–75%

―――――――――――――― *Strength Training: Upper Body* ――――――――――

CHOOSE ONE EXERCISE FOR EACH BODY PART:

Sets and Reps:

Beginner:
Sets: 1
Reps: 8–10

Intermediate:
Sets: 2
Reps: 10–12

Advanced:
Sets: 3
Reps 12–15

Chest
- Flyes on Pec Machine
- Chest Press on Bench Using Body Bar or Smith Machine
- Dumbbell Presses Over Exercise Ball
- Floor Push-Ups*

Back
- Lat Pull-Downs
- One-Arm Kneeling Rows
- Bent-Over Body Bar Rows
- Arm Pull-Downs*

Biceps
- Biceps Curls Using Dumbbells
- Seated One-Arm Biceps Curls

- Cable Biceps Curls
- Isometric Biceps Curls*

Triceps
- Triceps Extension Pull-Downs
- One-Arm Overhead Triceps Extension
- Lying Triceps Extension
- Triceps Wall Push-Ups*

Shoulders
- Angled One-Arm Side Raises
- Overhead Presses Using Dumbbells
- Reverse Flyes on Ball Using Dumbbells
- Reverse Flyes*

*Equipment-Free Exercises

―――――――――――――――― *Core* ―――――――――――――――

EXERCISE	FITNESS LEVEL	SETS	REPS
Back Extension on Exercise Ball	Beginner	1	8–10
	Intermediate	2	10–12
	Advanced	3	10–15
Cycle Rotations	Beginner	1	8–10
	Intermediate	2	10–12
	Advanced	3	12–15
Sitting Leg Lifts	Beginner	1	8–10
	Intermediate	2	10–12
	Advanced	3	10–15

―――――――――――――――― *Stretch* ―――――――――――――――

EXERCISE	SETS	HOLD
Hamstring Stretch: Single Leg Knee to Chest	3	15–60 Seconds
Piriformis Stretch	3	15–60 Seconds
Spinal Twist	3	15–60 Seconds

WEIGHT LOSS: WEEK THREE/ DAY 7
OPTIONAL: REST DAY

Aerobic

EXERCISE OPTIONS:	TIME:
Walking/Treadmill/Swimming/Biking/ Elliptical, Stairmaster/Aerobic Video	15 Minutes Heart Rate Goal: Between 65%–75%

Core

EXERCISE	FITNESS LEVEL	SETS	REPS
Isometric Squeezes	Beginner	1	8–10
	Intermediate	2	10–12
	Advanced	3	10–15
Kegels	Beginner	1	8–10
	Intermediate	2	10–12
	Advanced	3	12–15
Pelvic Tilts	Beginner	1	8–10
	Intermediate	2	10–12
	Advanced	3	10–15

Stretch

EXERCISE	SETS	HOLD
Hamstring Stretch: Single Leg Knee to Chest	3	15–60 Seconds
Hyper-Arch on Exercise Ball	3	15–60 Seconds
One Leg Forward Flexion	3	15–60 Seconds

WEIGHT LOSS: WEEK FOUR/ DAY 1

— Aerobic —

EXERCISE OPTIONS:	TIME:
Walking/Treadmill/Swimming/Biking/ Elliptical, Stairmaster/Aerobic Video	35 Minutes Heart Rate Goal: Between 65%–75%

— Core —

EXERCISE	FITNESS LEVEL	SETS	REPS
Ball Crunches	Beginner	1	8–10
	Intermediate	2	10–12
	Advanced	3	10–15
Lateral Side Drops on Ball	Beginner	1	8–10
	Intermediate	2	10–12
	Advanced	3	12–15
Reverse Leg Lifts with Ankle Weights	Beginner	1	8–10
	Intermediate	2	10–12
	Advanced	3	10–15

— Stretch —

EXERCISE	SETS	HOLD
Hamstring Stretch: Single Leg Knee to Chest	3	15–60 Seconds
Piriformis Stretch	3	15–60 Seconds
Spinal Twist	3	15–60 Seconds

WEIGHT LOSS: WEEK FOUR/ DAY 2

— Aerobic —

EXERCISE OPTIONS:	TIME:
Walking/Treadmill/Swimming/Biking/ Elliptical, Stairmaster/Aerobic	15 Minutes Heart Rate Goal: Between 65%–75%

———————————— *Strength Training: Lower Body* ————————————

CHOOSE ONE EXERCISE FOR EACH BODY PART:

SETS AND REPS:

Beginner:
Sets: 1
Reps: 8–10

Intermediate:
Sets: 2
Reps: 10–12

Advanced:
Sets: 3
Reps: 12–15

Glutes and Hips
- Plié Squats
- Dumbbell Squats
- Squats on Smith Machine
- Reverse Lunges*

Front of Legs
- Leg Extensions Using Ankle Weights
- Seated Leg Extension
- Inner Thigh Squats (Froggies)*
- Lying Bent Knee Leg Lifts*

Back of Legs
- Standing Hamstring Curls Using Ankle Weights

- Hamstring Curls Using Ankle Weights Over Bench, Chair or Ball
- Machine Hamstring Curls
- Standing Hamstring Curls*

Calves
- Standing Heel Raises Using Dumbbells
- Machine Heel Raises
- Heel Raises*

*Equipment-Free Exercise

———————————— *Core* ————————————

EXERCISE	FITNESS LEVEL	SETS	REPS
Quadruped Using Ankle Weights	Beginner	1	8–10
	Intermediate	2	10–12
	Advanced	3	10–15
Crunches on Exercise Bench Using Resistance Ball	Beginner	1	8–10
	Intermediate	2	10–12
	Advanced	3	12–15
Pelvic Tilts	Beginner	1	8–10
	Intermediate	2	10–12
	Advanced	3	10–15

———————————— *Stretch* ————————————

EXERCISE	SETS	HOLD
Hamstring Stretch: Single Leg Knee to Chest	3	15–60 Seconds
Quadriceps Stretch: Side-Lying Bent-Leg Stretch	3	15–60 Seconds
Hyper-Arch on Exercise Ball	3	15–60 Seconds

WEIGHT LOSS: WEEK FOUR/ DAY 3

Aerobic

EXERCISE OPTIONS:	TIME:
Walking/Treadmill/Swimming/Biking/ Elliptical, Stairmaster/Aerobic Video	35 Minutes Heart Rate Goal: Between 65%–75%

Core

EXERCISE	FITNESS LEVEL	SETS	REPS
Reverse Leg Lifts with Ankle Weights	Beginner	1	8–10
	Intermediate	2	10–12
	Advanced	3	10–15
Plank or Modified Plank	Beginner	1	8–10
	Intermediate	2	10–12
	Advanced	3	12–15
Lateral Drops on Exercise Ball	Beginner	1	8–10
	Intermediate	2	10–12
	Advanced	3	10–15

Stretch

EXERCISE	SETS	HOLD
One Leg Forward Flexion	3	15–60 Seconds
Piriformis Stretch	3	15–60 Seconds
Spinal Twist	3	15–60 Seconds

WEIGHT LOSS: WEEK FOUR/ DAY 4

Aerobic

EXERCISE OPTIONS:	TIME:
Walking/Treadmill/Swimming/Biking/ Elliptical, Stairmaster/Aerobic	15 Minutes Heart Rate Goal: Between 65%–75%

Strength Training: Upper Body

CHOOSE ONE EXERCISE FOR EACH BODY PART:

SETS AND REPS:

Beginner:
Sets: 1
Reps: 8–10

Intermediate:
Sets: 2
Reps: 10–12

Advanced:
Sets: 3
Reps: 12–15

Chest
- Flyes on Pec Machine
- Chest Press on Bench Using Body Bar or Smith Machine
- Dumbbell Presses Over Exercise Ball
- Floor Push-Ups*

Back
- Lat Pull-Downs
- One-Arm Kneeling Rows
- Bent-Over Body Bar Rows
- Arm Pull-Downs*

Biceps
- Biceps Curls Using Dumbbells
- Seated One-Arm Biceps Curls
- Cable Biceps Curls
- Isometric Biceps Curls*

Triceps
- Triceps Extension Pull-Downs
- One-Arm Overhead Triceps Extension
- Lying Triceps Extension
- Triceps Wall Push-Ups*

Shoulders
- Angled One-Arm Side Raises
- Overhead Presses Using Dumbbells
- Reverse Flyes on Ball Using Dumbbells
- Reverse Flyes*

*Equipment-Free Exercises

Core

EXERCISE	FITNESS LEVEL	SETS	REPS
Classic Crunches*	Beginner	1	8–10
	Intermediate	2	10–12
	Advanced	3	10–15
Cycle Rotations	Beginner	1	8–10
	Intermediate	2	10–12
	Advanced	3	12–15
Quadruped Using Ankle Weights	Beginner	1	8–10
	Intermediate	2	10–12
	Advanced	3	10–15

Stretch

EXERCISE	SETS	HOLD
Hamstring Stretch: Single Leg Knee to Chest	3	15–60 Seconds
Hyper-Arch on Exercise Ball	3	15–60 Seconds
Biceps/Triceps Stretches	3	15–60 Seconds

WEIGHT LOSS: WEEK FOUR/ DAY 5

— *Aerobic* —

EXERCISE OPTIONS:	TIME:
Walking/Treadmill/Swimming/Biking/ Elliptical, Stairmaster/Aerobic Video	35 Minutes Heart Rate Goal: Between 65%–75%

— *Core* —

EXERCISE	FITNESS LEVEL	SETS	REPS
Isometric Squeezes	Beginner	1	8–10
	Intermediate	2	10–12
	Advanced	3	10–15
Kegels	Beginner	1	8–10
	Intermediate	2	10–12
	Advanced	3	12–15
Ball Crunches	Beginner	1	8–10
	Intermediate	2	10–12
	Advanced	3	10–15

— *Stretch* —

EXERCISE	SETS	HOLD
Spinal Twist	3	15–60 Seconds
Hyper-Arch on Exercise Ball	3	15–60 Seconds
Piriformis Stretch	3	15–60 Seconds

WEIGHT LOSS: WEEK FOUR/ DAY 6

— *Aerobic* —

EXERCISE OPTIONS:	TIME:
Walking/Treadmill/Swimming/Biking/ Elliptical, Stairmaster/Aerobic	15 Minutes Heart Rate Goal: Between 65%–75%

Strength Training: Lower Body

CHOOSE ONE EXERCISE FOR EACH BODY PART:

SETS AND REPS:

Beginner:
Sets: 1
Reps: 8–10

Intermediate:
Sets: 2
Reps: 10–12

Advanced:
Sets: 3
Reps 12–15

Glutes and Hips
- Side-Lying Leg Lifts Using Exercise Band
- Dumbbell Squats
- Single Leg Lunges Using Resistance Ball
- Stationary Lunges*

Front of Legs
- Leg Extensions Using Ankle Weights
- Seated Leg Extension
- Inner Thigh Ball Squeezes
- Lying Bent Knee Leg Lifts*

Back of Legs
- Standing Hamstring Curls Using Ankle Weights

- Hamstring Curls Using Ankle Weights Over Bench, Chair or Ball
- Machine Hamstring Curls
- Standing Hamstring Curls*

Calves
- Standing Heel Raises Using Dumbbells
- Machine Heel Raises
- Heel Raises*

*Equipment-Free Exercises

Core

EXERCISE	FITNESS LEVEL	SETS	REPS
Quadruped Using Ankle Weights	Beginner	1	8–10
	Intermediate	2	10–12
	Advanced	3	10–15
Crunches on Exercise Bench Using Resistance Ball	Beginner	1	8–10
	Intermediate	2	10–12
	Advanced	3	12–15
Pelvic Tilts	Beginner	1	8–10
	Intermediate	2	10–12
	Advanced	3	10–15

Stretch

EXERCISE	SETS	HOLD
Hamstring Stretch: Single Leg Knee to Chest	3	15–60 Seconds
Quadriceps Stretch: Side-Lying Bent-Leg Stretch	3	15–60 Seconds
Hyper-Arch on Exercise Ball	3	15–60 Seconds

WEIGHT LOSS: WEEK FOUR/ DAY 7
OPTIONAL: REST DAY

Aerobic

EXERCISE OPTIONS:	TIME:
Walking/Treadmill/Swimming/Biking/ Elliptical, Stairmaster/Aerobic Video	15 Minutes Heart Rate Goal: Between 65%–75%

Core

EXERCISE	FITNESS LEVEL	SETS	REPS
Isometric Squeezes	Beginner	1	8–10
	Intermediate	2	10–12
	Advanced	3	10–15
Kegels	Beginner	1	8–10
	Intermediate	2	10–12
	Advanced	3	12–15
Plank or Modified Plank	Beginner	1	8–10
	Intermediate	2	10–12
	Advanced	3	10–15

Stretch

EXERCISE	SETS	HOLD
Hamstring Stretch: Single Leg Knee to Chest	3	15–60 Seconds
Spinal Twist	3	15–60 Seconds
Piriformis Stretch	3	15–60 Seconds

WEIGHT LOSS: WEEK FIVE/ DAY 1

Aerobic

EXERCISE OPTIONS:	TIME:
Walking/Treadmill/Swimming/Biking/ Elliptical, Stairmaster/Aerobic Video	35 Minutes Heart Rate Goal: Between 65%–75%

Core

EXERCISE	FITNESS LEVEL	SETS	REPS
Classic Crunches	Beginner	1	8–10
	Intermediate	2	10–12
	Advanced	3	10–15
Cycle Rotations	Beginner	1	8–10
	Intermediate	2	10–12
	Advanced	3	12–15
Reverse Leg Lifts Using Ankle Weights	Beginner	1	8–10
	Intermediate	2	10–12
	Advanced	3	10–15

Stretch

EXERCISE	SETS	HOLD
Hamstring Stretch: Single Leg Knee to Chest	3	15–60 Seconds
Piriformis Stretch	3	15–60 Seconds
Spinal Twist	3	15–60 Seconds

WEIGHT LOSS: WEEK FIVE/ DAY 2

Aerobic

EXERCISE OPTIONS:	TIME:
Walking/Treadmill/Swimming/Biking/ Elliptical, Stairmaster/Aerobic	15 Minutes Heart Rate Goal: Between 65%–75%

Strength Training: Upper Body

CHOOSE ONE EXERCISE FOR EACH BODY PART:

SETS AND REPS:

Beginner:
Sets: 1
Reps: 8–10

Intermediate:
Sets: 2
Reps: 10–12

Advanced:
Sets: 3
Reps: 12–15

Chest
- Ball Push-Ups
- Chest Press on Bench Using Body Bar or Smith Machine
- Dumbbell Presses Over Exercise Ball
- Wall Push-Ups*

Back
- Lat Pull-Downs
- One-Arm Kneeling Rows
- Machine Assisted Pull-Ups
- Back Rows*

Biceps
- Biceps Curls Using Dumbbells
- Body Bar Biceps Curls
- Cable Biceps Curls
- Isometric Biceps Curls*

Triceps
- Triceps Extensions Pull-Downs
- One-Arm Overhead Triceps Extension
- Lying Triceps Extension
- Triceps V-Backs*

Shoulders
- Side Arm Raises Using Dumbbells
- Overhead Presses Using Dumbbells
- Reverse Flyes on Ball Using Dumbbells
- Reverse Flyes*

*Equipment-Free Exercises

Core

EXERCISE	FITNESS LEVEL	SETS	REPS
Ball Crunches	Beginner	1	8–10
	Intermediate	2	10–12
	Advanced	3	10–15
Lateral Side Drops on Ball	Beginner	1	8–10
	Intermediate	2	10–12
	Advanced	3	12–15
Sitting Leg Lifts	Beginner	1	8–10
	Intermediate	2	10–12
	Advanced	3	10–15

Stretch

EXERCISE	SETS	HOLD
Hamstring Stretch: Single Leg Knee to Chest	3	15–60 Seconds
Piriformis Stretch	3	15–60 Seconds
Biceps/Triceps Stretches	3	15–60 Seconds

WEIGHT LOSS: WEEK FIVE/ DAY 3

Aerobic

EXERCISE OPTIONS:	TIME:
Walking/Treadmill/Swimming/Biking/ Elliptical, Stairmaster/Aerobic Video	35 Minutes Heart Rate Goal: Between 65%–75%

Core

EXERCISE	FITNESS LEVEL	SETS	REPS
Reverse Leg Lifts with Ankle Weights	Beginner	1	8–10
	Intermediate	2	10–12
	Advanced	3	10–15
Cycle Rotations	Beginner	1	8–10
	Intermediate	2	10–12
	Advanced	3	12–15
Back Extensions on Exercise Ball	Beginner	1	8–10
	Intermediate	2	10–12
	Advanced	3	10–15

Stretch

EXERCISE	SETS	HOLD
One Leg Forward Flexion	3	15–60 Seconds
Hyper-Arch on Exercise Ball	3	15–60 Seconds
Spinal Twist	3	15–60 Seconds

WEIGHT LOSS: WEEK FIVE/ DAY 4

Aerobic

EXERCISE OPTIONS:	TIME:
Walking/Treadmill/Swimming/Biking/ Elliptical, Stairmaster/Aerobic	15 Minutes Heart Rate Goal: Between 65%–75%

Strength Training: Lower Body

CHOOSE ONE EXERCISE FOR EACH BODY PART:

SETS AND REPS:

Beginner:
Sets: 1
Reps: 8–10

Intermediate:
Sets: 2
Reps: 10–12

Advanced:
Sets: 3
Reps: 12–15

Glutes and Hips
- Ball Squats
- Side-Lying Leg Lifts Using Exercise Band
- Reverse Lunges Using Ankle Weights
- Sit Downs*

Front of Legs
- Plié Squats Against Ball
- Seated Leg Extension
- Leg Extensions Using Ankle Weights
- Lying Bent Knee Leg Lifts*

Back of Legs
- Standing Hamstring Curls Using Ankle Weights

- Hamstring Curls Using Ankle Weights Over Bench, Chair or Ball
- Machine Hamstring Curls
- Standing Hamstring Curls*

Calves
- Standing Heel Raises Using Dumbbells
- Machine Heel Raises
- Heel Raises*

*Equipment-Free Exercise

Core

EXERCISE	FITNESS LEVEL	SETS	REPS
Plank or Modified Plank	Beginner	1	8–10
	Intermediate	2	10–12
	Advanced	3	10–15
Ball Crunches	Beginner	1	8–10
	Intermediate	2	10–12
	Advanced	3	12–15
Kegels	Beginner	1	8–10
	Intermediate	2	10–12
	Advanced	3	10–15

Stretch

EXERCISE	SETS	HOLD
Hamstring Stretch: Single Leg Knee to Chest	3	15–60 Seconds
Quadriceps Stretch: Side-Lying Bent-Leg Stretch	3	15–60 Seconds
Hyper-Arch on Exercise Ball	3	15–60 Seconds

WEIGHT LOSS: WEEK FIVE/ DAY 5

Aerobic

EXERCISE OPTIONS:	TIME:
Walking/Treadmill/Swimming/Biking/ Elliptical, Stairmaster/Aerobic Video	35 Minutes Heart Rate Goal: Between 65%–75%

Core

EXERCISE	FITNESS LEVEL	SETS	REPS
Isometric Squeezes	Beginner	1	8–10
	Intermediate	2	10–12
	Advanced	3	10–15
Pelvic Tilts	Beginner	1	8–10
	Intermediate	2	10–12
	Advanced	3	12–15
Crunches on Flat Bench Using Resistance Ball	Beginner	1	8–10
	Intermediate	2	10–12
	Advanced	3	10–15

Stretch

EXERCISE	SETS	HOLD
Spinal Twist	3	15–60 Seconds
Hyper-Arch on Exercise Ball	3	15–60 Seconds
Piriformis Stretch	3	15–60 Seconds

WEIGHT LOSS: WEEK FIVE/ DAY 6

Aerobic

EXERCISE OPTIONS:	TIME:
Walking/Treadmill/Swimming/Biking/ Elliptical, Stairmaster/Aerobic	15 Minutes Heart Rate Goal: Between 65%–75%

―――――――――――― *Strength Training: Upper Body* ――――――――――――

CHOOSE ONE EXERCISE FOR EACH BODY PART:

SETS AND REPS:

Beginner:
Sets: 1
Reps: 8–10

Intermediate:
Sets: 2
Reps: 10–12

Advanced:
Sets: 3
Reps: 12–15

Chest
- Chest Flyes Using Dumbbells on Flat Bench
- Chest Press on Bench Using Body Bar or Smith Machine
- Dumbbell Presses Over Exercise Ball
- Floor Push-Ups*

Back
- Lat Pull-Downs
- One-Arm Kneeling Rows
- Bent-Over Body Bar Rows
- Arm Pull-Downs*

Biceps
- Biceps Curls Using Dumbbells
- Seated One-Arm Biceps Curls
- Cable Biceps Curls
- Isometric Biceps Curls*

Triceps
- Triceps Extension Pull-Downs
- One-Arm Overhead Triceps Extension
- Lying Triceps Extension
- Triceps Wall Push-Ups*

Shoulders
- Angled One-Arm Side Raises
- Overhead Presses Using Dumbbells
- Reverse Flyes on Ball Using Dumbbells
- Reverse Flyes*

*Equipment-Free Exercises

――――――――――――――――――― *Core* ―――――――――――――――――――

EXERCISE	FITNESS LEVEL	SETS	REPS
Back Extensions on Exercise Ball	Beginner	1	8–10
	Intermediate	2	10–12
	Advanced	3	10–15
Cycle Rotations	Beginner	1	8–10
	Intermediate	2	10–12
	Advanced	3	12–15
Sitting Leg Lifts	Beginner	1	8–10
	Intermediate	2	10–12
	Advanced	3	10–15

――――――――――――――――――― *Stretch* ―――――――――――――――――――

EXERCISE	SETS	HOLD
One Leg Forward Flexion	3	15–60 Seconds
Piriformis Stretch	3	15–60 Seconds
Spinal Twist	3	15–60 Seconds

WEIGHT LOSS: WEEK FIVE/ DAY 7
OPTIONAL: REST DAY

Aerobic

EXERCISE OPTIONS:	TIME:
Walking/Treadmill/Swimming/Biking/ Elliptical, Stairmaster/Aerobic Video	15 Minutes Heart Rate Goal: Between 65%–75%

Core

EXERCISE	FITNESS LEVEL	SETS	REPS
Leg Lifts	Beginner	1	8–10
	Intermediate	2	10–12
	Advanced	3	10–15
Kegels	Beginner	1	8–10
	Intermediate	2	10–12
	Advanced	3	12–15
Pelvic Tilts	Beginner	1	8–10
	Intermediate	2	10–12
	Advanced	3	10–15

Stretch

EXERCISE	SETS	HOLD
Hamstring Stretch: Single Leg Knee to Chest	3	15–60 Seconds
Hyper-Arch on Exercise Ball	3	15–60 Seconds
One Leg Forward Flexion	3	15–60 Seconds

WEIGHT LOSS: WEEK SIX/ DAY 1

Aerobic

EXERCISE OPTIONS:	TIME:
Walking/Treadmill/Swimming/Biking/ Elliptical, Stairmaster/Aerobic Video	40–45 Minutes Heart Rate Goal: Between 65%–75%

Core

EXERCISE	FITNESS LEVEL	SETS	REPS
Ball Crunches	Beginner	1	8–10
	Intermediate	2	10–12
	Advanced	3	10–15
Lateral Side Drops on Ball	Beginner	1	8–10
	Intermediate	2	10–12
	Advanced	3	12–15
Reverse Leg Lifts with Ankle Weights	Beginner	1	8–10
	Intermediate	2	10–12
	Advanced	3	10–15

Stretch

EXERCISE	SETS	HOLD
Hamstring Stretch: Single Leg Knee to Chest	3	15–60 Seconds
Piriformis Stretch	3	15–60 Seconds
Spinal Twist	3	15–60 Seconds

WEIGHT LOSS: WEEK SIX/ DAY 2

Aerobic

EXERCISE OPTIONS:	TIME:
Walking/Treadmill/Swimming/Biking/ Elliptical, Stairmaster/Aerobic	15 Minutes Heart Rate Goal: Between 65%–75%

--- *Strength Training: Lower Body* ---

CHOOSE ONE EXERCISE FOR EACH BODY PART:

SETS AND REPS:

Beginner:
Sets: 1
Reps: 8–10

Intermediate:
Sets: 2
Reps: 10–12

Advanced:
Sets: 3
Reps 12–15

Glutes and Hips
- Ball Squats
- Step-Ups Using Barbell or Dumbbells
- Squats on Smith Machine
- Reverse Lunges*

Front of Legs
- Leg Extensions Using Ankle Weights
- Seated Leg Extension
- Side-Lying Inner Thigh Lifts Using Ankle Weights
- Lying Bent Knee Leg Lifts*

Back of Legs
- Standing Hamstring Curls Using Ankle Weights

- Hamstring Curls Using Ankle Weights Over Bench, Chair or Ball
- Machine Hamstring Curls
- Standing Hamstring Curls*

Calves
- Standing Heel Raises Using Dumbbells
- Machine Heel Raises
- Heel Raises*

*Equipment-Free Exercises

--- *Core* ---

EXERCISE	FITNESS LEVEL	SETS	REPS
Leg Lifts	Beginner	1	8–10
	Intermediate	2	10–12
	Advanced	3	10–15
Crunches on Exercise Bench Using Resistance Ball	Beginner	1	8–10
	Intermediate	2	10–12
	Advanced	3	12–15
Pelvic Tilts	Beginner	1	8–10
	Intermediate	2	10–12
	Advanced	3	10–15

--- *Stretch* ---

EXERCISE	SETS	HOLD
One Leg Forward Flexion	3	15–60 Seconds
Quadriceps Stretch: Side-Lying Bent-Leg Stretch	3	15–60 Seconds
Hyper-Arch on Exercise Ball	3	15–60 Seconds

WEIGHT LOSS: WEEK SIX/ DAY 3

Aerobic

EXERCISE OPTIONS:	TIME:
Walking/Treadmill/Swimming/Biking/ Elliptical, Stairmaster/Aerobic Video	40–45 Minutes Heart Rate Goal: Between 65%–75%

Core

EXERCISE	FITNESS LEVEL	SETS	REPS
Reverse Leg Lifts Using Ankle Weights	Beginner	1	8–10
	Intermediate	2	10–12
	Advanced	3	10–15
Plank or Modified Plank	Beginner	1	8–10
	Intermediate	2	10–12
	Advanced	3	12–15
Lateral Drops on Exercise Ball	Beginner	1	8–10
	Intermediate	2	10–12
	Advanced	3	10–15

Stretch

EXERCISE	SETS	HOLD
One Leg Forward Flexion	3	15–60 Seconds
Piriformis Stretch	3	15–60 Seconds
Spinal Twist	3	15–60 Seconds

WEIGHT LOSS: WEEK SIX/ DAY 4

Aerobic

EXERCISE OPTIONS:	TIME:
Walking/Treadmill/Swimming/Biking/ Elliptical, Stairmaster/Aerobic	15 Minutes Heart Rate Goal: Between 65%–75%

Strength Training: Upper Body

CHOOSE ONE EXERCISE FOR EACH BODY PART:

SETS AND REPS:

Beginner:
Sets: 1
Reps: 8–10

Intermediate:
Sets: 2
Reps: 10–12

Advanced:
Sets: 3
Reps 12–15

Chest
- Flyes on Pec Machine
- Chest Press on Bench Using Body Bar or Smith Machine
- Dumbbell Presses Over Exercise Ball
- Presses*

Back
- Lat Pull-Downs
- Seated Low Rows
- Bent-Over Body Bar Rows
- Arm Pull-Downs

Biceps
- Biceps Curls Using Dumbbells
- Body Bar Biceps Curls
- Cable Biceps Curls
- Isometric Biceps Curls*

Triceps
- Triceps Extensions Pull-Downs
- One-Arm Overhead Triceps Extension
- Lying Triceps Extension
- Overhead Triceps Extension*

Shoulders
- One Arm Front Delt Lifts Using Dumbbells
- Shoulder Press Machine
- Reverse Flyes on Ball Using Dumbbells
- Overhead Presses

*Equipment-Free Exercises

Core

EXERCISE	FITNESS LEVEL	SETS	REPS
Classic Crunches*	Beginner	1	8–10
	Intermediate	2	10–12
	Advanced	3	10–15
Cycle Rotations	Beginner	1	8–10
	Intermediate	2	10–12
	Advanced	3	12–15
Quadruped Using Ankle Weights	Beginner	1	8–10
	Intermediate	2	10–12
	Advanced	3	10–15

Stretch

EXERCISE	SETS	HOLD
Hamstring Stretch: Single Leg Knee to Chest	3	15–60 Seconds
Hyper-Arch on Exercise Ball	3	15–60 Seconds
Biceps/Triceps Stretches	3	15–60 Seconds

WEIGHT LOSS: WEEK SIX/ DAY 5

Aerobic

EXERCISE OPTIONS:	TIME:
Walking/Treadmill/Swimming/Biking/ Elliptical, Stairmaster/Aerobic Video	40–45 Minutes Heart Rate Goal: Between 65%–75%

Core

EXERCISE	FITNESS LEVEL	SETS	REPS
Back Extensions on Exercise Ball	Beginner	1	8–10
	Intermediate	2	10–12
	Advanced	3	10–15
Kegels	Beginner	1	8–10
	Intermediate	2	10–12
	Advanced	3	12–15
Ball Crunches	Beginner	1	8–10
	Intermediate	2	10–12
	Advanced	3	10–15

Stretch

EXERCISE	SETS	HOLD
Spinal Twist	3	15–60 Seconds
Hyper-Arch on Exercise Ball	3	15–60 Seconds
Piriformis Stretch	3	15–60 Seconds

WEIGHT LOSS: WEEK SIX/ DAY 6

Aerobic

EXERCISE OPTIONS:	TIME:
Walking/Treadmill/Swimming/Biking/ Elliptical, Stairmaster/Aerobic	15 Minutes Heart Rate Goal: Between 65%–75%

Strength Training: Lower Body

CHOOSE ONE EXERCISE FOR EACH BODY PART:

SETS AND REPS:

Beginner:
Sets: 1
Reps: 8–10

Intermediate:
Sets: 2
Reps: 10–12

Advanced:
Sets: 3
Reps 12–15

Glutes and Hips
- Side-Lying Leg Lifts Using Exercise Band
- Step-Ups Using Barbell or Dumbbells
- Single Leg Lunges Using Resistance Ball
- Stationary Lunges*

Front of Legs
- Leg Extensions Using Ankle Weights
- Seated Leg Extension
- Inner Thigh Ball Squeezes
- Lying Bent Knee Leg Lifts*

Back of Legs
- Standing Hamstring Curls Using Ankle Weights

- Hamstring Curls Using Ankle Weights Over Bench, Chair or Ball
- Machine Hamstring Curls
- Standing Hamstring Curls*

Calves
- Standing Heel Raises Using Dumbbells
- Machine Heel Raises
- Heel Raises*

*Equipment-Free Exercise

Core

EXERCISE	FITNESS LEVEL	SETS	REPS
Quadruped Using Ankle Weights	Beginner	1	8–10
	Intermediate	2	10–12
	Advanced	3	10–15
Crunches on Exercise Bench Using Resistance Ball	Beginner	1	8–10
	Intermediate	2	10–12
	Advanced	3	12–15
Pelvic Tilts	Beginner	1	8–10
	Intermediate	2	10–12
	Advanced	3	10–15

Stretch

EXERCISE	SETS	HOLD
One-Leg Forward Flexion	3	15–60 Seconds
Quadriceps Stretch: Side-Lying Bent-Leg Stretch	3	15–60 Seconds
Hyper-Arch on Exercise Ball	3	15–60 Seconds

WEIGHT LOSS: WEEK SIX/ DAY 7
OPTIONAL: REST DAY

Aerobic

EXERCISE OPTIONS:	TIME:
Walking/Treadmill/Swimming/Biking/ Elliptical, Stairmaster/Aerobic Video	15 Minutes Heart Rate Goal: Between 65%–75%

Core

EXERCISE	FITNESS LEVEL	SETS	REPS
Isometric Squeezes	Beginner	1	8–10
	Intermediate	2	10–12
	Advanced	3	10–15
Kegels	Beginner	1	8–10
	Intermediate	2	10–12
	Advanced	3	12–15
Plank or Modified Plank	Beginner	1	8–10
	Intermediate	2	10–12
	Advanced	3	10–15

Stretch

EXERCISE	SETS	HOLD
Hamstring Stretch: Single Leg Knee to Chest	3	15–60 Seconds
Spinal Twist	3	15–60 Seconds
Piriformis Stretch	3	15–60 Seconds

Anti-Aging Workout System 2
Goal: Increase Strength, Tone, and Firm

INCREASE STRENGTH: WEEK ONE/ DAY 1

Aerobic

EXERCISE OPTIONS:	TIME:
Walking/Treadmill/Swimming/Biking/ Elliptical, Stairmaster/Aerobic	7 Minutes Heart Rate Goal: Between 65%–75%

Strength Training: Upper Body

CHOOSE TWO EXERCISES FOR EACH BODY PART:

SETS AND REPS:

Beginner:
Sets: 1
Reps: 8–10

Intermediate:
Sets: 2
Reps: 10–12

Advanced:
Sets: 3
Reps: 12–15

Chest
• Ball Push-Ups
• Chest Press on Bench Using Body Bar or Smith Machine
• Dumbbell Presses Over Exercise Ball
• Wall Push-Ups*

Back
• Lat Pull-Downs
• One-Arm Kneeling Rows
• Machine Assisted Pull-Ups
• Back Rows*

Biceps
• Biceps Curls Using Dumbbells
• Body Bar Biceps Curls
• Cable Biceps Curls
• Isometric Biceps Curls*

Triceps
• Triceps Extensions Pull-Downs
• One-Arm Overhead Triceps Extension
• Lying Triceps Extension
• Triceps V-Backs*

Shoulders
• Side Arm Raises Using Dumbbells
• Overhead Presses Using Dumbbells
• Reverse Flyes on Ball Using Dumbbells
• Reverse Flyes*

*Equipment-Free Exercises

Core

EXERCISE	FITNESS LEVEL	SETS	REPS
Ball Crunches	Beginner	1	8–10
	Intermediate	2	10–12
	Advanced	3	10–15
Lateral Side Drops on Ball	Beginner	1	8–10
	Intermediate	2	10–12
	Advanced	3	12–15
Sitting Leg Lifts	Beginner	1	8–10
	Intermediate	2	10–12
	Advanced	3	10–15

Stretch

EXERCISE	SETS	HOLD
Hamstring Stretch: Single Leg Knee to Chest	3	15–60 Seconds
Piriformis Stretch	3	15–60 Seconds
Biceps/Triceps Stretches	3	15–60 Seconds

INCREASE STRENGTH: WEEK ONE/ DAY 2

Aerobic

EXERCISE OPTIONS:	TIME:
Walking/Treadmill/Swimming/Biking/ Elliptical, Stairmaster/Aerobic Video	25 Minutes Heart Rate Goal: Between 65%–75%

Core

EXERCISE	FITNESS LEVEL	SETS	REPS
Reverse Leg Lifts with Ankle Weights	Beginner	1	8–10
	Intermediate	2	10–12
	Advanced	3	10–15
Cycle Rotations	Beginner	1	8–10
	Intermediate	2	10–12
	Advanced	3	12–15
Back Extensions on Exercise Ball	Beginner	1	8–10
	Intermediate	2	10–12
	Advanced	3	10–15

Stretch

EXERCISE	SETS	HOLD
One Leg Forward Flexion	3	15–60 Seconds
Hyper-Arch on Exercise Ball	3	15–60 Seconds
Spinal Twist	3	15–60 Seconds

INCREASE STRENGTH: WEEK ONE/ DAY 3

Aerobic

EXERCISE OPTIONS:	TIME:
Walking/Treadmill/Swimming/Biking/ Elliptical, Stairmaster/Aerobic	7 Minutes Heart Rate Goal: Between 65%–75%

Strength Training: Lower Body

CHOOSE TWO EXERCISES FOR EACH BODY PART:

SETS AND REPS:

Beginner:
Sets: 1
Reps: 8–10

Intermediate:
Sets: 2
Reps: 10–12

Advanced:
Sets: 3
Reps: 12–15

Glutes and Hips
• Ball Squats
• Side-Lying Leg Lifts Using Exercise Band
• Reverse Lunges Using Ankle Weights
• Sit Downs*

Front of Legs
• Plié Squats Against Ball
• Seated Leg Extension
• Leg Extensions Using Ankle Weights
• Lying Bent Knee Leg Lifts*

Back of Legs
• Standing Hamstring Curls Using Ankle Weights

• Hamstring Curls Using Ankle Weights Over Bench, Chair or Ball
• Machine Hamstring Curls
• Standing Hamstring Curls*

Calves
• Standing Heel Raises Using Dumbbells
• Machine Heel Raises
• Heel Raises*

*Equipment-Free Exercise

Core

EXERCISE	FITNESS LEVEL	SETS	REPS
Plank or Modified Plank	Beginner	1	8–10
	Intermediate	2	10–12
	Advanced	3	10–15
Ball Crunches	Beginner	1	8–10
	Intermediate	2	10–12
	Advanced	3	12–15
Kegels	Beginner	1	8–10
	Intermediate	2	10–12
	Advanced	3	10–15

Stretch

EXERCISE	SETS	HOLD
Hamstring Stretch: Single Leg Knee to Chest	3	15–60 Seconds
Quadriceps Stretch: Side-Lying Bent-Leg Stretch	3	15–60 Seconds
Hyper-Arch on Exercise Ball	3	15–60 Seconds

INCREASE STRENGTH: WEEK ONE/ DAY 4

Aerobic

EXERCISE OPTIONS:	TIME:
Walking/Treadmill/Swimming/Biking/ Elliptical, Stairmaster/Aerobic Video	25 Minutes Heart Rate Goal: Between 65%–75%

Core

EXERCISE	FITNESS LEVEL	SETS	REPS
Isometric Squeezes	Beginner	1	8–10
	Intermediate	2	10–12
	Advanced	3	10–15
Pelvic Tilts	Beginner	1	8–10
	Intermediate	2	10–12
	Advanced	3	12–15
Crunches on Flat Bench Using Resistance Ball	Beginner	1	8–10
	Intermediate	2	10–12
	Advanced	3	10–15

Stretch

EXERCISE	SETS	HOLD
Spinal Twist	3	15–60 Seconds
Hyper-Arch on Exercise Ball	3	15–60 Seconds
Piriformis Stretch	3	15–60 Seconds

INCREASE STRENGTH: WEEK ONE/ DAY 5

———————— Aerobic ————————

EXERCISE OPTIONS:	TIME:
Walking/Treadmill/Swimming/Biking/ Elliptical, Stairmaster/Aerobic	7 Minutes Heart Rate Goal: Between 65%–75%

———— Strength Training: Upper Body ————

CHOOSE TWO EXERCISES FOR EACH BODY PART:

SETS AND REPS:

Beginner:
Sets: 1
Reps: 8–10

Intermediate:
Sets: 2
Reps: 10–12

Advanced:
Sets: 3
Reps: 12–15

Chest
- Chest Flyes Using Dumbbells on Flat Bench
- Chest Press on Bench Using Body Bar or Smith Machine
- Dumbbell Presses Over Exercise Ball
- Floor Push-Ups*

Back
- Lat Pull-Downs
- One-Arm Kneeling Rows
- Bent-Over Body Bar Rows
- Arm Pull-Downs*

Biceps
- Biceps Curls Using Dumbbells

- Seated One-Arm Biceps Curls
- Cable Biceps Curls
- Isometric Biceps Curls*

Triceps
- Triceps Extension Pull-Downs
- One-Arm Overhead Triceps Extension
- Lying Triceps Extension
- Triceps Wall Push-Ups*

Shoulders
- Angled One-Arm Side Raises
- Overhead Presses Using Dumbbells
- Reverse Flyes on Ball Using Dumbbells
- Reverse Flyes*

*Equipment-Free Exercises

———————— Core ————————

EXERCISE	FITNESS LEVEL	SETS	REPS
Back Extensions on Exercise Ball	Beginner	1	8–10
	Intermediate	2	10–12
	Advanced	3	10–15
Cycle Rotations	Beginner	1	8–10
	Intermediate	2	10–12
	Advanced	3	12–15
Sitting Leg Lifts	Beginner	1	8–10
	Intermediate	2	10–12
	Advanced	3	10–15

Stretch

EXERCISE	SETS	HOLD
One Leg Forward Flexion	3	15–60 Seconds
Piriformis Stretch	3	15–60 Seconds
Spinal Twist	3	15–60 Seconds

INCREASE STRENGTH: WEEK ONE/ DAY 6
OPTIONAL: REST DAY

Aerobic

EXERCISE OPTIONS:	TIME:
Walking/Treadmill/Swimming/Biking/ Elliptical, Stairmaster/Aerobic Video	25 Minutes Heart Rate Goal: Between 65%–75%

Core

EXERCISE	FITNESS LEVEL	SETS	REPS
Leg Lifts	Beginner	1	8–10
	Intermediate	2	10–12
	Advanced	3	10–15
Kegels	Beginner	1	8–10
	Intermediate	2	10–12
	Advanced	3	12–15
Pelvic Tilts	Beginner	1	8–10
	Intermediate	2	10–12
	Advanced	3	10–15

Stretch

EXERCISE	SETS	HOLD
Hamstring Stretch: Single Leg Knee to Chest	3	15–60 Seconds
Hyper-Arch on Exercise Ball	3	15–60 Seconds
One Leg Forward Flexion	3	15–60 Seconds

INCREASE STRENGTH: WEEK ONE/ DAY 7

Aerobic

EXERCISE OPTIONS:	TIME:
Walking/Treadmill/Swimming/Biking/ Elliptical, Stairmaster/Aerobic	7 Minutes Heart Rate Goal: Between 65%–75%

Strength Training: Lower Body

CHOOSE TWO EXERCISES FOR EACH BODY PART:

SETS AND REPS:

Beginner:
Sets: 1
Reps: 8–10

Intermediate:
Sets: 2
Reps: 10–12

Advanced:
Sets: 3
Reps 12–15

Glutes and Hips
- Ball Squats
- Step-Ups Using Barbell or Dumbbells
- Squats on Smith Machine
- Reverse Lunges*

Front of Legs
- Leg Extensions Using Ankle Weights
- Seated Leg Extension
- Side-Lying Inner Thigh Lifts Using Ankle Weights
- Lying Bent Knee Leg Lifts*

Back of Legs
- Standing Hamstring Curls Using Ankle Weights
- Hamstring Curls Using Ankle Weights Over Bench, Chair or Ball
- Machine Hamstring Curls
- Standing Hamstring Curls*

Calves
- Standing Heel Raises Using Dumbbells
- Machine Heel Raises
- Heel Raises*

*Equipment-Free Exercises

―――――――――――――――――― *Core* ――――――――――――――――――

EXERCISE	FITNESS LEVEL	SETS	REPS
Leg Lifts	Beginner	1	8–10
	Intermediate	2	10–12
	Advanced	3	10–15
Crunches on Exercise Bench Using Resistance Ball	Beginner	1	8–10
	Intermediate	2	10–12
	Advanced	3	12–15
Pelvic Tilts	Beginner	1	8–10
	Intermediate	2	10–12
	Advanced	3	10–15

―――――――――――――――――― *Stretch* ――――――――――――――――――

EXERCISE	SETS	HOLD
One Leg Forward Flexion	3	15–60 Seconds
Quadriceps Stretch: Side-Lying Bent-Leg Stretch	3	15–60 Seconds
Hyper-Arch on Exercise Ball	3	15–60 Seconds

INCREASE STRENGTH: WEEK TWO/ DAY 1

Aerobic

EXERCISE OPTIONS:	TIME:
Walking/Treadmill/Swimming/Biking/ Elliptical, Stairmaster/Aerobic	7 Minutes Heart Rate Goal: Between 65%–75%

Strength Training: Upper Body

CHOOSE TWO EXERCISES FOR EACH BODY PART:

SETS AND REPS:

Beginner:
Sets: 1
Reps: 8–10

Intermediate:
Sets: 2
Reps: 10–12

Advanced:
Sets: 3
Reps 12–15

Chest
- Flyes on Pec Machine
- Chest Press on Bench Using Body Bar or Smith Machine
- Dumbbell Presses Over Exercise Ball
- Presses*

Back
- Lat Pull-Downs
- Seated Low Rows
- Bent-Over Body Bar Rows
- Arm Pull-Downs

Biceps
- Biceps Curls Using Dumbbells
- Body Bar Biceps Curls
- Cable Biceps Curls
- Isometric Biceps Curls*

Triceps
- Triceps Extensions Pull-Downs
- One-Arm Overhead Triceps Extension
- Lying Triceps Extension
- Overhead Triceps Extension*

Shoulders
- One Arm Front Delt Lifts Using Dumbbells
- Shoulder Press Machine
- Reverse Flyes on Ball Using Dumbbells
- Overhead Presses

*Equipment-Free Exercises

Core

EXERCISE	FITNESS LEVEL	SETS	REPS
Classic Crunches*	Beginner	1	8–10
	Intermediate	2	10–12
	Advanced	3	10–15
Cycle Rotations	Beginner	1	8–10
	Intermediate	2	10–12
	Advanced	3	12–15
Quadruped Using Ankle Weights	Beginner	1	8–10
	Intermediate	2	10–12
	Advanced	3	10–15

Stretch

EXERCISE	SETS	HOLD
Hamstring Stretch: Single Leg Knee to Chest	3	15–60 Seconds
Hyper-Arch on Exercise Ball	3	15–60 Seconds
Biceps/Triceps Stretches	3	15–60 Seconds

INCREASE STRENGTH: WEEK TWO/ DAY 2

Aerobic

EXERCISE OPTIONS:	TIME:
Walking/Treadmill/Swimming/Biking/ Elliptical, Stairmaster/Aerobic Video	25 Minutes Heart Rate Goal: Between 65%–75%

Core

EXERCISE	FITNESS LEVEL	SETS	REPS
Ball Crunches	Beginner	1	8–10
	Intermediate	2	10–12
	Advanced	3	10–15
Lateral Side Drops on Ball	Beginner	1	8–10
	Intermediate	2	10–12
	Advanced	3	12–15
Reverse Leg Lifts with Ankle Weights	Beginner	1	8–10
	Intermediate	2	10–12
	Advanced	3	10–15

Stretch

EXERCISE	SETS	HOLD
Hamstring Stretch: Single Leg Knee to Chest	3	15–60 Seconds
Piriformis Stretch	3	15–60 Seconds
Spinal Twist	3	15–60 Seconds

INCREASE STRENGTH: WEEK TWO/ DAY 3

Aerobic

EXERCISE OPTIONS:	TIME:
Walking/Treadmill/Swimming/Biking/ Elliptical, Stairmaster/Aerobic	7 Minutes Heart Rate Goal: Between 65%–75%

Strength Training: Lower Body

CHOOSE TWO EXERCISES FOR EACH BODY PART:

SETS AND REPS:

Beginner:
Sets: 1
Reps: 8–10

Intermediate:
Sets: 2
Reps: 10–12

Advanced:
Sets: 3
Reps 12–15

Glutes and Hips
- Ball Squats
- Step-Ups Using Barbell or Dumbbells
- Squats on Smith Machine
- Reverse Lunges*

Front of Legs
- Leg Extensions Using Ankle Weights
- Seated Leg Extension
- Side-Lying Inner Thigh Lifts Using Ankle Weights
- Lying Bent Knee Leg Lifts*

Back of Legs
- Standing Hamstring Curls Using Ankle Weights

- Hamstring Curls Using Ankle Weights Over Bench, Chair or Ball
- Machine Hamstring Curls
- Standing Hamstring Curls*

Calves
- Standing Heel Raises Using Dumbbells
- Machine Heel Raises
- Heel Raises*

*Equipment-Free Exercises

Core

EXERCISE	FITNESS LEVEL	SETS	REPS
Leg Lifts	Beginner	1	8–10
	Intermediate	2	10–12
	Advanced	3	10–15
Crunches on Exercise Bench Using Resistance Ball	Beginner	1	8–10
	Intermediate	2	10–12
	Advanced	3	12–15
Pelvic Tilts	Beginner	1	8–10
	Intermediate	2	10–12
	Advanced	3	10–15

Stretch

EXERCISE	SETS	HOLD
One Leg Forward Flexion	3	15–60 Seconds
Quadriceps Stretch: Side-Lying Bent-Leg Stretch	3	15–60 Seconds
Hyper-Arch on Exercise Ball	3	15–60 Seconds

INCREASE STRENGTH: WEEK TWO/ DAY 4

Aerobic

EXERCISE OPTIONS:	TIME:
Walking/Treadmill/Swimming/Biking/ Elliptical, Stairmaster/Aerobic Video	25 Minutes Heart Rate Goal: Between 65%–75%

Core

EXERCISE	FITNESS LEVEL	SETS	REPS
Reverse Leg Lifts Using Ankle Weights	Beginner	1	8–10
	Intermediate	2	10–12
	Advanced	3	10–15
Plank or Modified Plank	Beginner	1	8–10
	Intermediate	2	10–12
	Advanced	3	12–15
Lateral Drops on Exercise Ball	Beginner	1	8–10
	Intermediate	2	10–12
	Advanced	3	10–15

Stretch

EXERCISE	SETS	HOLD
One Leg Forward Flexion	3	15–60 Seconds
Piriformis Stretch	3	15–60 Seconds
Spinal Twist	3	15–60 Seconds

INCREASE STRENGTH: WEEK TWO/ DAY 5

Aerobic

EXERCISE OPTIONS:	TIME:
Walking/Treadmill/Swimming/Biking/ Elliptical, Stairmaster/Aerobic	7 Minutes Heart Rate Goal: Between 65%–75%

Strength Training: Upper Body

CHOOSE TWO EXERCISES FOR EACH BODY PART:

SETS AND REPS:

Beginner:
Sets: 1
Reps: 8–10

Intermediate:
Sets: 2
Reps: 10–12

Advanced:
Sets: 3
Reps 12–15

Chest
- Ball Push-Ups
- Chest Press Using Body Bar/Smith Machine
- Dumbbell Presses on Ball
- Wall Push-Ups*

Back
- Lat Pull Downs
- One-Arm Kneeling Rows
- Machine Assisted Pull-Ups
- Back Rows*

Biceps
- Biceps Curls Using Dumbbells
- Body Bar Biceps Curls
- Cable Biceps Curls
- Isometric Biceps Curls*

Triceps
- Triceps Extension Pull-Downs
- One-Arm Overhead Triceps Extension
- Lying Triceps Extension
- Triceps V-Backs*

Shoulders
- One Arm Front Delt Lifts Using Dumbbells
- Shoulder Press Machine
- Reverse Flyes on Ball Using Dumbbells
- Overhead Presses*

*Equipment-Free Exercises

Core

EXERCISE	FITNESS LEVEL	SETS	REPS
Ball Crunches	Beginner	1	8–10
	Intermediate	2	10–12
	Advanced	3	10–15
Lateral Side Drops on Ball	Beginner	1	8–10
	Intermediate	2	10–12
	Advanced	3	12–15
Sitting Leg Lifts	Beginner	1	8–10
	Intermediate	2	10–12
	Advanced	3	10–15

Stretch

EXERCISE	SETS	HOLD
Hamstring Stretch: Single Leg Knee to Chest	3	15–60 Seconds
Piriformis Stretch	3	15–60 Seconds
Biceps/Triceps Stretches	3	15–60 Seconds

INCREASE STRENGTH: WEEK TWO/ DAY 6
OPTIONAL: REST DAY

Aerobic

EXERCISE OPTIONS:	TIME:
Walking/Treadmill/Swimming/Biking/ Elliptical, Stairmaster/Aerobic Video	25 Minutes Heart Rate Goal: Between 65%–75%

Core

EXERCISE	FITNESS LEVEL	SETS	REPS
Back Extensions on Exercise Ball	Beginner	1	8–10
	Intermediate	2	10–12
	Advanced	3	10–15
Kegels	Beginner	1	8–10
	Intermediate	2	10–12
	Advanced	3	12–15
Ball Crunches	Beginner	1	8–10
	Intermediate	2	10–12
	Advanced	3	10–15

Stretch

EXERCISE	SETS	HOLD
Spinal Twist	3	15–60 Seconds
Hyper-Arch on Exercise Ball	3	15–60 Seconds
Piriformis Stretch	3	15–60 Seconds

INCREASE STRENGTH: WEEK TWO/ DAY 7

Aerobic

EXERCISE OPTIONS:	TIME:
Walking/Treadmill/Swimming/Biking/ Elliptical, Stairmaster/Aerobic	7 Minutes Heart Rate Goal: Between 65%–75%

Strength Training: Lower Body

CHOOSE TWO EXERCISES FOR EACH BODY PART

SETS AND REPS:

Beginner:
Sets: 1
Reps: 8–10

Intermediate:
Sets: 2
Reps: 10–12

Advanced:
Sets: 3
Reps 12–15

Glutes and Hips
- Side-Lying Leg Lifts Using Exercise Band
- Step-Ups Using Barbell or Dumbbells
- Single Leg Lunges Using Resistance Ball
- Stationary Lunges*

Front of Legs
- Leg Extensions Using Ankle Weights
- Seated Leg Extension
- Inner Thigh Ball Squeezes
- Lying Bent Knee Leg Lifts*

Back of Legs
- Standing Hamstring Curls Using Ankle Weights
- Hamstring Curls Using Ankle Weights Over Bench, Chair or Ball
- Machine Hamstring Curls
- Standing Hamstring Curls*

Calves
- Standing Heel Raises Using Dumbbells
- Machine Heel Raises
- Heel Raises*

*Equipment-Free Exercise

Core

EXERCISE	FITNESS LEVEL	SETS	REPS
Quadruped Using Ankle Weights	Beginner	1	8–10
	Intermediate	2	10–12
	Advanced	3	10–15
Crunches on Exercise Bench Using Resistance Ball	Beginner	1	8–10
	Intermediate	2	10–12
	Advanced	3	12–15
Pelvic Tilts	Beginner	1	8–10
	Intermediate	2	10–12
	Advanced	3	10–15

Stretch

EXERCISE	SETS	HOLD
One-Leg Forward Flexion	3	15–60 Seconds
Quadriceps Stretch: Side-Lying Bent-Leg Stretch	3	15–60 Seconds
Hyper-Arch on Exercise Ball	3	15–60 Seconds

INCREASE STRENGTH: WEEK THREE/ DAY 1

Aerobic

EXERCISE OPTIONS:	TIME:
Walking/Treadmill/Swimming/Biking/ Elliptical, Stairmaster/Aerobic	7 Minutes Heart Rate Goal: Between 65%–75%

Strength Training: Upper Body

CHOOSE TWO EXERCISES FOR EACH BODY PART:

SETS AND REPS:

Beginner:
Sets: 1
Reps: 8–10

Intermediate:
Sets: 2
Reps: 10–12

Advanced:
Sets: 3
Reps 12–15

Chest
• Ball Push-Ups
• Chest Press Using Body Bar/Smith Machine
• Dumbbell Presses on Ball
• Wall Push-Ups*

Back
• Lat Pull Downs
• One-Arm Kneeling Rows
• Machine Assisted Pull-Ups
• Back Rows*

Biceps
• Biceps Curls Using Dumbbells
• Body Bar Biceps Curls

• Cable Biceps Curls
• Isometric Biceps Curls*

Triceps
• Triceps Extension Pull-Downs
• One-Arm Overhead Triceps Extension
• Lying Triceps Extension
• Triceps V-Backs*

Shoulders
• One Arm Front Delt Lifts Using Dumbbells
• Shoulder Press Machine
• Reverse Flyes on Ball Using Dumbbells
• Overhead Presses*

*Equipment-Free Exercises

Core

EXERCISE	FITNESS LEVEL	SETS	REPS
Ball Crunches	Beginner	1	8–10
	Intermediate	2	10–12
	Advanced	3	10–15
Lateral Side Drops on Ball	Beginner	1	8–10
	Intermediate	2	10–12
	Advanced	3	12–15
Sitting Leg Lifts	Beginner	1	8–10
	Intermediate	2	10–12
	Advanced	3	10–15

Stretch

EXERCISE	SETS	HOLD
Hamstring Stretch: Single Leg Knee to Chest	3	15–60 Seconds
Piriformis Stretch	3	15–60 Seconds
Biceps/Triceps Stretches	3	15–60 Seconds

INCREASE STRENGTH: WEEK THREE/ DAY 2

Aerobic

EXERCISE OPTIONS:	TIME:
Walking/Treadmill/Swimming/Biking/ Elliptical, Stairmaster/Aerobic Video	30 Minutes Heart Rate Goal: Between 65%–75%

Core

EXERCISE	FITNESS LEVEL	SETS	REPS
Reverse Leg Lifts with Ankle Weights	Beginner	1	8–10
	Intermediate	2	10–12
	Advanced	3	10–15
Cycle Rotations	Beginner	1	8–10
	Intermediate	2	10–12
	Advanced	3	12–15
Back Extensions on Exercise Ball	Beginner	1	8–10
	Intermediate	2	10–12
	Advanced	3	10–15

Stretch

EXERCISE	SETS	HOLD
One Leg Forward Flexion	3	15–60 Seconds
Hyper-Arch on Exercise Ball	3	15–60 Seconds
Spinal Twist	3	15–60 Seconds

INCREASE STRENGTH: WEEK THREE/ DAY 3

Aerobic

EXERCISE OPTIONS:	TIME:
Walking/Treadmill/Swimming/Biking/ Elliptical, Stairmaster/Aerobic	7 Minutes Heart Rate Goal: Between 65%–75%

Strength Training: Lower Body

CHOOSE ONE EXERCISE FOR EACH BODY PART:

SETS AND REPS:

Beginner:
Sets: 1
Reps: 8–10

Intermediate:
Sets: 2
Reps: 10–12

Advanced:
Sets: 3
Reps 12–15

Glutes and Hips
- Ball Squats
- Side-Lying Leg Lifts Using Exercise Band
- Reverse Lunges Using Ankle Weights
- Sit Downs*

Front of Legs
- Plié Squats Against Ball
- Seated Leg Extension
- Leg Extensions Using Ankle Weights
- Lying Bent Knee Leg Lifts*

Back of Legs
- Standing Hamstring Curls Using Ankle Weights

- Hamstring Curls Using Ankle Weights Over Bench, Chair or Ball
- Machine Hamstring Curls
- Standing Hamstring Curls*

Calves
- Standing Heel Raises Using Dumbbells
- Machine Heel Raises
- Heel Raises*

*Equipment-Free Exercise

Core

EXERCISE	FITNESS LEVEL	SETS	REPS
Plank or Modified Plank	Beginner	1	8–10
	Intermediate	2	10–12
	Advanced	3	10–15
Ball Crunches	Beginner	1	8–10
	Intermediate	2	10–12
	Advanced	3	12–15
Kegels	Beginner	1	8–10
	Intermediate	2	10–12
	Advanced	3	10–15

―――――――――――――――――― *Stretch* ――――――――――――――――――

EXERCISE	SETS	HOLD
Hamstring Stretch: Single Leg Knee to Chest	3	15–60 Seconds
Quadriceps Stretch: Side-Lying Bent-Leg Stretch	3	15–60 Seconds
Hyper-Arch on Exercise Ball	3	15–60 Seconds

INCREASE STRENGTH: WEEK THREE/ DAY 4

―――――――――――――――――― *Aerobic* ――――――――――――――――――

EXERCISE OPTIONS:	TIME:
Walking/Treadmill/Swimming/Biking/ Elliptical, Stairmaster/Aerobic Video	30 Minutes Heart Rate Goal: Between 65%–75%

―――――――――――――――――― *Core* ――――――――――――――――――

EXERCISE	FITNESS LEVEL	SETS	REPS
Isometric Squeezes	Beginner	1	8–10
	Intermediate	2	10–12
	Advanced	3	10–15
Pelvic Tilts	Beginner	1	8–10
	Intermediate	2	10–12
	Advanced	3	12–15
Crunches on Flat Bench Using Resistance Ball	Beginner	1	8–10
	Intermediate	2	10–12
	Advanced	3	10–15

―――――――――――――――――― *Stretch* ――――――――――――――――――

EXERCISE	SETS	HOLD
Spinal Twist	3	15–60 Seconds
One Leg Forward Flexion	3	15–60 Seconds
Hyper-Arch on Exercise Ball	3	15–60 Seconds

INCREASE STRENGTH: WEEK THREE/ DAY 5

Aerobic

EXERCISE OPTIONS:	TIME:
Walking/Treadmill/Swimming/Biking/ Elliptical, Stairmaster/Aerobic	7 Minutes Heart Rate Goal: Between 65%–75%

Strength Training: Upper Body

CHOOSE TWO EXERCISES FOR EACH BODY PART:

SETS AND REPS:

Beginner:
Sets: 1
Reps: 8–10

Intermediate:
Sets: 2
Reps: 10–12

Advanced:
Sets: 3
Reps 12–15

Chest
- Flyes on Pec Machine
- Chest Press on Bench Using Body Bar or Smith Machine
- Dumbbell Presses Over Exercise Ball
- Floor Push-Ups*

Back
- Lat Pull-Downs
- One-Arm Kneeling Rows
- Bent-Over Body Bar Rows
- Arm Pull-Downs*

Biceps
- Biceps Curls Using Dumbbells
- Seated One-Arm Biceps Curls

- Cable Biceps Curls
- Isometric Biceps Curls*

Triceps
- Triceps Extension Pull-Downs
- One-Arm Overhead Triceps Extension
- Lying Triceps Extension
- Triceps Wall Push-Ups*

Shoulders
- Angled One-Arm Side Raises
- Overhead Presses Using Dumbbells
- Reverse Flyes on Ball Using Dumbbells
- Reverse Flyes*

*Equipment-Free Exercises

Core

EXERCISE	FITNESS LEVEL	SETS	REPS
Back Extension on Exercise Ball	Beginner	1	8–10
	Intermediate	2	10–12
	Advanced	3	10–15
Cycle Rotations	Beginner	1	8–10
	Intermediate	2	10–12
	Advanced	3	12–15
Sitting Leg Lifts	Beginner	1	8–10
	Intermediate	2	10–12
	Advanced	3	10–15

─────────────────── *Stretch* ───────────────────

EXERCISE	SETS	HOLD
Hamstring Stretch: Single Leg Knee to Chest	3	15–60 Seconds
Piriformis Stretch	3	15–60 Seconds
Spinal Twist	3	15–60 Seconds

INCREASE STRENGTH: WEEK THREE/ DAY 6
OPTIONAL: REST DAY

─────────────────── *Aerobic* ───────────────────

EXERCISE OPTIONS:	TIME:
Walking/Treadmill/Swimming/Biking/ Elliptical, Stairmaster/Aerobic Video	30 Minutes Heart Rate Goal: Between 65%–75%

─────────────────── *Core* ───────────────────

EXERCISE	FITNESS LEVEL	SETS	REPS
Isometric Squeezes	Beginner	1	8–10
	Intermediate	2	10–12
	Advanced	3	10–15
Kegels	Beginner	1	8–10
	Intermediate	2	10–12
	Advanced	3	12–15
Pelvic Tilts	Beginner	1	8–10
	Intermediate	2	10–12
	Advanced	3	10–15

Stretch

EXERCISE	SETS	HOLD
Hamstring Stretch: Single Leg Knee to Chest	3	15–60 Seconds
Hyper-Arch on Exercise Ball	3	15–60 Seconds
One Leg Forward Flexion	3	15–60 Seconds

INCREASE STRENGTH: WEEK THREE/ DAY 7

Aerobic

EXERCISE OPTIONS:	TIME:
Walking/Treadmill/Swimming/Biking/ Elliptical, Stairmaster/Aerobic	7 Minutes Heart Rate Goal: Between 65%–75%

Strength Training: Lower Body

CHOOSE TWO EXERCISES FOR EACH BODY PART:

SETS AND REPS:

Beginner:
Sets: 1
Reps: 8–10

Intermediate:
Sets: 2
Reps: 10–12

Advanced:
Sets: 3
Reps 12–15

Glutes and Hips
- Ball Squats
- Step-Ups Using Barbell or Dumbbells
- Squats on Smith Machine
- Reverse Lunges*

Front of Legs
- Leg Extensions Using Ankle Weights
- Seated Leg Extension
- Side-Lying Inner Thigh Lifts Using Ankle Weights
- Lying Bent Knee Leg Lifts*

Back of Legs
- Standing Hamstring Curls Using Ankle Weights

- Hamstring Curls Using Ankle Weights Over Bench, Chair or Ball
- Machine Hamstring Curls
- Standing Hamstring Curls*

Calves
- Standing Heel Raises Using Dumbbells
- Machine Heel Raises
- Heel Raises*

*Equipment-Free Exercises

Core

EXERCISE	FITNESS LEVEL	SETS	REPS
Leg Lifts	Beginner	1	8–10
	Intermediate	2	10–12
	Advanced	3	10–15
Crunches on Exercise Bench Using Resistance Ball	Beginner	1	8–10
	Intermediate	2	10–12
	Advanced	3	12–15
Pelvic Tilts	Beginner	1	8–10
	Intermediate	2	10–12
	Advanced	3	10–15

Stretch

EXERCISE	SETS	HOLD
One Leg Forward Flexion	3	15–60 Seconds
Quadriceps Stretch: Side-Lying Bent-Leg Stretch	3	15–60 Seconds
Hyper-Arch on Exercise Ball	3	15–60 Seconds

INCREASE STRENGTH: WEEK FOUR/ DAY 1

Aerobic

EXERCISE OPTIONS:	TIME:
Walking/Treadmill/Swimming/Biking/ Elliptical, Stairmaster/Aerobic	7 Minutes Heart Rate Goal: Between 65%–75%

Strength Training: Upper Body

CHOOSE TWO EXERCISES FOR EACH BODY PART:

SETS AND REPS:

Beginner:
Sets: 1
Reps: 8–10

Intermediate:
Sets: 2
Reps: 10–12

Advanced:
Sets: 3
Reps: 12–15

Chest
- Flyes on Pec Machine
- Chest Press on Bench Using Body Bar or Smith Machine
- Dumbbell Presses Over Exercise Ball
- Floor Push-Ups*

Back
- Lat Pull-Downs
- One-Arm Kneeling Rows
- Bent-Over Body Bar Rows
- Arm Pull-Downs*

Biceps
- Biceps Curls Using Dumbbells
- Seated One-Arm Biceps Curls

- Cable Biceps Curls
- Isometric Biceps Curls*

Triceps
- Triceps Extension Pull-Downs
- One-Arm Overhead Triceps Extension
- Lying Triceps Extension
- Triceps Wall Push-Ups*

Shoulders
- Angled One-Arm Side Raises
- Overhead Presses Using Dumbbells
- Reverse Flyes on Ball Using Dumbbells
- Reverse Flyes*

*Equipment-Free Exercises

Core

EXERCISE	FITNESS LEVEL	SETS	REPS
Classic Crunches*	Beginner	1	8–10
	Intermediate	2	10–12
	Advanced	3	10–15
Cycle Rotations	Beginner	1	8–10
	Intermediate	2	10–12
	Advanced	3	12–15
Quadruped Using Ankle Weights	Beginner	1	8–10
	Intermediate	2	10–12
	Advanced	3	10–15

Stretch

EXERCISE	SETS	HOLD
Hamstring Stretch: Single Leg Knee to Chest	3	15–60 Seconds
Hyper-Arch on Exercise Ball	3	15–60 Seconds
Biceps/Triceps Stretches	3	15–60 Seconds

INCREASE STRENGTH: WEEK FOUR/DAY 2

Aerobic

EXERCISE OPTIONS:	TIME:
Walking/Treadmill/Swimming/Biking/ Elliptical, Stairmaster/Aerobic Video	30 Minutes Heart Rate Goal: Between 65%–75%

Core

EXERCISE	FITNESS LEVEL	SETS	REPS
Isometric Squeezes	Beginner	1	8–10
	Intermediate	2	10–12
	Advanced	3	10–15
Kegels	Beginner	1	8–10
	Intermediate	2	10–12
	Advanced	3	12–15
Ball Crunches	Beginner	1	8–10
	Intermediate	2	10–12
	Advanced	3	10–15

Stretch

EXERCISE	SETS	HOLD
Spinal Twist	3	15–60 Seconds
Hyper-Arch on Exercise Ball	3	15–60 Seconds
Piriformis Stretch	3	15–60 Seconds

INCREASE STRENGTH: WEEK FOUR/DAY 3

Aerobic

EXERCISE OPTIONS:	TIME:
Walking/Treadmill/Swimming/Biking/ Elliptical, Stairmaster/Aerobic	7 Minutes Heart Rate Goal: Between 65%–75%

Strength Training: Lower Body

CHOOSE TWO EXERCISES FOR EACH BODY PART:

SETS AND REPS:

Beginner:
Sets: 1
Reps: 8–10

Intermediate:
Sets: 2
Reps: 10–12

Advanced:
Sets: 3
Reps 12–15

Glutes and Hips
- Side-Lying Leg Lifts Using Exercise Band
- Dumbbell Squats
- Single Leg Lunges Using Resistance Ball
- Stationary Lunges*

Front of Legs
- Leg Extensions Using Ankle Weights
- Seated Leg Extension
- Inner Thigh Ball Squeezes
- Lying Bent Knee Leg Lifts*

Back of Legs
- Standing Hamstring Curls Using Ankle Weights
- Hamstring Curls Using Ankle Weights Over Bench, Chair or Ball
- Machine Hamstring Curls
- Standing Hamstring Curls*

Calves
- Standing Heel Raises Using Dumbbells
- Machine Heel Raises
- Heel Raises*

*Equipment-Free Exercises

Core

EXERCISE	FITNESS LEVEL	SETS	REPS
Quadruped Using Ankle Weights	Beginner	1	8–10
	Intermediate	2	10–12
	Advanced	3	10–15
Crunches on Exercise Bench Using Resistance Ball	Beginner	1	8–10
	Intermediate	2	10–12
	Advanced	3	12–15
Pelvic Tilts	Beginner	1	8–10
	Intermediate	2	10–12
	Advanced	3	10–15

―――――――――――――― *Stretch* ――――――――――――――

EXERCISE	SETS	HOLD
Hamstring Stretch: Single Leg Knee to Chest	3	15–60 Seconds
Quadriceps Stretch: Side-Lying Bent-Leg Stretch	3	15–60 Seconds
Hyper-Arch on Exercise Ball	3	15–60 Seconds

INCREASE STRENGTH: WEEK FOUR/DAY 4

―――――――――――――― *Aerobic* ――――――――――――――

EXERCISE OPTIONS:	TIME:
Walking/Treadmill/Swimming/Biking/ Elliptical, Stairmaster/Aerobic Video	35 Minutes Heart Rate Goal: Between 65%–75%

―――――――――――――― *Core* ――――――――――――――

EXERCISE	FITNESS LEVEL	SETS	REPS
Isometric Squeezes	Beginner	1	8–10
	Intermediate	2	10–12
	Advanced	3	10–15
Kegels	Beginner	1	8–10
	Intermediate	2	10–12
	Advanced	3	12–15
Plank or Modified Plank	Beginner	1	8–10
	Intermediate	2	10–12
	Advanced	3	10–15

―――――――――――――― *Stretch* ――――――――――――――

EXERCISE	SETS	HOLD
Hamstring Stretch: Single Leg Knee to Chest	3	15–60 Seconds
Spinal Twist	3	15–60 Seconds
Piriformis Stretch	3	15–60 Seconds

INCREASE STRENGTH: WEEK FOUR/DAY 5

Aerobic

EXERCISE OPTIONS:	TIME:
Walking/Treadmill/Swimming/Biking/ Elliptical, Stairmaster/Aerobic	7 Minutes Heart Rate Goal: Between 65%–75%

Strength Training: Upper Body

CHOOSE TWO EXERCISES FOR EACH BODY PART:

SETS AND REPS:

Beginner:
Sets: 1
Reps: 8–10

Intermediate:
Sets: 2
Reps: 10–12

Advanced:
Sets: 3
Reps: 12–15

Chest
- Ball Push-Ups
- Chest Press on Bench Using Body Bar or Smith Machine
- Dumbbell Presses Over Exercise Ball
- Wall Push-Ups*

Back
- Lat Pull-Downs
- One-Arm Kneeling Rows
- Machine Assisted Pull-Ups
- Back Rows*

Biceps
- Biceps Curls Using Dumbbells
- Body Bar Biceps Curls

- Cable Biceps Curls
- Isometric Biceps Curls*

Triceps
- Triceps Extensions Pull-Downs
- One-Arm Overhead Triceps Extension
- Lying Triceps Extension
- Triceps V-Backs*

Shoulders
- Side Arm Raises Using Dumbbells
- Overhead Presses Using Dumbbells
- Reverse Flyes on Ball Using Dumbbells
- Reverse Flyes*

*Equipment-Free Exercises

Core

EXERCISE	FITNESS LEVEL	SETS	REPS
Ball Crunches	Beginner	1	8–10
	Intermediate	2	10–12
	Advanced	3	10–15
Lateral Side Drops on Ball	Beginner	1	8–10
	Intermediate	2	10–12
	Advanced	3	12–15
Sitting Leg Lifts	Beginner	1	8–10
	Intermediate	2	10–12
	Advanced	3	10–15

Stretch

EXERCISE	SETS	HOLD
Hamstring Stretch: Single Leg Knee to Chest	3	15–60 Seconds
Piriformis Stretch	3	15–60 Seconds
Biceps/Triceps Stretches	3	15–60 Seconds

INCREASE STRENGTH: WEEK FOUR/DAY 6
OPTIONAL: REST DAY

Aerobic

EXERCISE OPTIONS:	TIME:
Walking/Treadmill/Swimming/Biking/ Elliptical, Stairmaster/Aerobic Video	20 Minutes Heart Rate Goal: Between 65%–75%

Core

EXERCISE	FITNESS LEVEL	SETS	REPS
Reverse Leg Lifts with Ankle Weights	Beginner	1	8–10
	Intermediate	2	10–12
	Advanced	3	10–15
Cycle Rotations	Beginner	1	8–10
	Intermediate	2	10–12
	Advanced	3	12–15
Back Extensions on Exercise Ball	Beginner	1	8–10
	Intermediate	2	10–12
	Advanced	3	10–15

Stretch

EXERCISE	SETS	HOLD
One Leg Forward Flexion	3	15–60 Seconds
Hyper-Arch on Exercise Ball	3	15–60 Seconds
Spinal Twist	3	15–60 Seconds

INCREASE STRENGTH: WEEK FOUR/DAY 7

Aerobic

EXERCISE OPTIONS:	TIME:
Walking/Treadmill/Swimming/Biking/ Elliptical, Stairmaster/Aerobic	7 Minutes Heart Rate Goal: Between 65%–75%

Strength Training: Lower Body

CHOOSE TWO EXERCISES FOR EACH BODY PART:

SETS AND REPS:

Beginner:
Sets: 1
Reps: 8–10

Intermediate:
Sets: 2
Reps: 10–12

Advanced:
Sets: 3
Reps: 12–15

Glutes and Hips
- Plié Squats
- Dumbbell Squats
- Squats on Smith Machine
- Reverse Lunges*

Front of Legs
- Leg Extensions Using Ankle Weights
- Seated Leg Extension
- Inner Thigh Squats (Froggies)*
- Lying Bent Knee Leg Lifts*

Back of Legs
- Standing Hamstring Curls Using Ankle Weights

- Hamstring Curls Using Ankle Weights Over Bench, Chair or Ball
- Machine Hamstring Curls
- Standing Hamstring Curls*

Calves
- Standing Heel Raises Using Dumbbells
- Machine Heel Raises
- Heel Raises*

*Equipment-Free Exercise

————————————— *Core* —————————————

EXERCISE	FITNESS LEVEL	SETS	REPS
Quadruped Using Ankle Weights	Beginner	1	8–10
	Intermediate	2	10–12
	Advanced	3	10–15
Crunches on Exercise Bench Using Resistance Ball	Beginner	1	8–10
	Intermediate	2	10–12
	Advanced	3	12–15
Pelvic Tilts	Beginner	1	8–10
	Intermediate	2	10–12
	Advanced	3	10–15

————————————— *Stretch* —————————————

EXERCISE	SETS	HOLD
Hamstring Stretch: Single Leg Knee to Chest	3	15–60 Seconds
Quadriceps Stretch: Side-Lying Bent-Leg Stretch	3	15–60 Seconds
Hyper Arch on Exercise Ball	3	15–60 Seconds

INCREASE STRENGTH: WEEK FIVE/ DAY 1

Aerobic

EXERCISE OPTIONS:	TIME:
Walking/Treadmill/Swimming/Biking/ Elliptical, Stairmaster/Aerobic	8 Minutes Heart Rate Goal: Between 65%–75%

Strength Training: Upper Body

CHOOSE TWO EXERCISES FOR EACH BODY PART:

SETS AND REPS:

Beginner:
Sets: 1
Reps: 8–10

Intermediate:
Sets: 2
Reps: 10–12

Advanced:
Sets: 3
Reps: 12–15

Chest
- Ball Push-Ups
- Chest Press on Bench Using Body Bar or Smith Machine
- Dumbbell Presses Over Exercise Ball
- Wall Push-Ups*

Back
- Lat Pull-Downs
- One-Arm Kneeling Rows
- Machine Assisted Pull-Ups
- Back Rows*

Biceps
- Biceps Curls Using Dumbbells
- Body Bar Biceps Curls

- Cable Biceps Curls
- Isometric Biceps Curls*

Triceps
- Triceps Extensions Pull-Downs
- One-Arm Overhead Triceps Extension
- Lying Triceps Extension
- Triceps V-Backs*

Shoulders
- Side Arm Raises Using Dumbbells
- Overhead Presses Using Dumbbells
- Reverse Flyes on Ball Using Dumbbells
- Reverse Flyes*

*Equipment-Free Exercises

Core

EXERCISE	FITNESS LEVEL	SETS	REPS
Ball Crunches	Beginner	1	8–10
	Intermediate	2	10–12
	Advanced	3	10–15
Lateral Side Drops on Ball	Beginner	1	8–10
	Intermediate	2	10–12
	Advanced	3	12–15
Sitting Leg Lifts	Beginner	1	8–10
	Intermediate	2	10–12
	Advanced	3	10–15

———————————————— *Stretch* ————————————————

EXERCISE	SETS	HOLD
Hamstring Stretch: Single Leg Knee to Chest	3	15–60 Seconds
Piriformis Stretch	3	15–60 Seconds
Biceps/Triceps Stretches	3	15–60 Seconds

INCREASE STRENGTH: WEEK FIVE/DAY 2

———————————————— *Aerobic* ————————————————

EXERCISE OPTIONS:	TIME:
Walking/Treadmill/Swimming/Biking/ Elliptical, Stairmaster/Aerobic Video	30 Minutes Heart Rate Goal: Between 65%–75%

———————————————— *Core* ————————————————

EXERCISE	FITNESS LEVEL	SETS	REPS
Reverse Leg Lifts with Ankle Weights	Beginner	1	8–10
	Intermediate	2	10–12
	Advanced	3	10–15
Cycle Rotations	Beginner	1	8–10
	Intermediate	2	10–12
	Advanced	3	12–15
Back Extensions on Exercise Ball	Beginner	1	8–10
	Intermediate	2	10–12
	Advanced	3	10–15

———————————————— *Stretch* ————————————————

EXERCISE	SETS	HOLD
One Leg Forward Flexion	3	15–60 Seconds
Hyper-Arch on Exercise Ball	3	15–60 Seconds
Spinal Twist	3	15–60 Seconds

INCREASE STRENGTH: WEEK FIVE/ DAY 3

Aerobic

EXERCISE OPTIONS:	TIME:
Walking/Treadmill/Swimming/Biking/ Elliptical, Stairmaster/Aerobic	7 Minutes Heart Rate Goal: Between 65%–75%

Strength Training: Lower Body

CHOOSE TWO EXERCISES FOR EACH BODY PART:

SETS AND REPS:

Beginner:
Sets: 1
Reps: 8–10

Intermediate:
Sets: 2
Reps: 10–12

Advanced:
Sets: 3
Reps: 12–15

Glutes and Hips
- Ball Squats
- Side-Lying Leg Lifts Using Exercise Band
- Reverse Lunges Using Ankle Weights
- Sit Downs*

Front of Legs
- Plié Squats Against Ball
- Seated Leg Extension
- Leg Extensions Using Ankle Weights
- Lying Bent Knee Leg Lifts*

Back of Legs
- Standing Hamstring Curls Using Ankle Weights
- Hamstring Curls Using Ankle Weights Over Bench, Chair or Ball
- Machine Hamstring Curls
- Standing Hamstring Curls*

Calves
- Standing Heel Raises Using Dumbbells
- Machine Heel Raises
- Heel Raises*

*Equipment-Free Exercise

Core

EXERCISE	FITNESS LEVEL	SETS	REPS
Plank or Modified Plank	Beginner	1	8–10
	Intermediate	2	10–12
	Advanced	3	10–15
Ball Crunches	Beginner	1	8–10
	Intermediate	2	10–12
	Advanced	3	12–15
Kegels	Beginner	1	8–10
	Intermediate	2	10–12
	Advanced	3	10–15

Stretch

EXERCISE	SETS	HOLD
Hamstring Stretch: Single Leg Knee to Chest	3	15–60 Seconds
Quadriceps Stretch: Side-Lying Bent-Leg Stretch	3	15–60 Seconds
Hyper-Arch on Exercise Ball	3	15–60 Seconds

INCREASE STRENGTH: WEEK FIVE/ DAY 4

Aerobic

EXERCISE OPTIONS:	TIME:
Walking/Treadmill/Swimming/Biking/ Elliptical, Stairmaster/Aerobic Video	30 Minutes Heart Rate Goal: Between 65%–75%

Core

EXERCISE	FITNESS LEVEL	SETS	REPS
Isometric Squeezes	Beginner	1	8–10
	Intermediate	2	10–12
	Advanced	3	10–15
Pelvic Tilts	Beginner	1	8–10
	Intermediate	2	10–12
	Advanced	3	12–15
Crunches on Flat Bench Using Resistance Ball	Beginner	1	8–10
	Intermediate	2	10–12
	Advanced	3	10–15

Stretch

EXERCISE	SETS	HOLD
Spinal Twist	3	15–60 Seconds
Hyper-Arch on Exercise Ball	3	15–60 Seconds
Piriformis Stretch	3	15–60 Seconds

INCREASE STRENGTH: WEEK FIVE/ DAY 5

Aerobic

EXERCISE OPTIONS:	TIME:
Walking/Treadmill/Swimming/Biking/ Elliptical, Stairmaster/Aerobic	7 Minutes Heart Rate Goal: Between 65%–75%

Strength Training: Upper Body

CHOOSE TWO EXERCISES FOR EACH BODY PART:

SETS AND REPS:

Beginner:
Sets: 1
Reps: 8–10

Intermediate:
Sets: 2
Reps: 10–12

Advanced:
Sets: 3
Reps: 12–15

Chest
• Chest Flyes Using Dumbbells on Flat Bench
• Chest Press on Bench Using Body Bar or Smith Machine
• Dumbbell Presses Over Exercise Ball
• Floor Push-Ups*

Back
• Lat Pull-Downs
• One-Arm Kneeling Rows
• Bent-Over Body Bar Rows
• Arm Pull-Downs*

Biceps
• Biceps Curls Using Dumbbells

• Seated One-Arm Biceps Curls
• Cable Biceps Curls
• Isometric Biceps Curls*

Triceps
• Triceps Extension Pull-Downs
• One-Arm Overhead Triceps Extension
• Lying Triceps Extension
• Triceps Wall Push-Ups*

Shoulders
• Angled One-Arm Side Raises
• Overhead Presses Using Dumbbells
• Reverse Flyes on Ball Using Dumbbells
• Reverse Flyes*

*Equipment-Free Exercises

Core

EXERCISE	FITNESS LEVEL	SETS	REPS
Back Extensions on Exercise Ball	Beginner	1	8–10
	Intermediate	2	10–12
	Advanced	3	10–15
Cycle Rotations	Beginner	1	8–10
	Intermediate	2	10–12
	Advanced	3	12–15
Sitting Leg Lifts	Beginner	1	8–10
	Intermediate	2	10–12
	Advanced	3	10–15

Stretch

EXERCISE	SETS	HOLD
One Leg Forward Flexion	3	15–60 Seconds
Piriformis Stretch	3	15–60 Seconds
Spinal Twist	3	15–60 Seconds

INCREASE STRENGTH: WEEK FIVE/ DAY 6
OPTIONAL: REST DAY

Aerobic

EXERCISE OPTIONS:	TIME:
Walking/Treadmill/Swimming/Biking/ Elliptical, Stairmaster/Aerobic Video	30 Minutes Heart Rate Goal: Between 65%–75%

Core

EXERCISE	FITNESS LEVEL	SETS	REPS
Leg Lifts	Beginner	1	8–10
	Intermediate	2	10–12
	Advanced	3	10–15
Kegels	Beginner	1	8–10
	Intermediate	2	10–12
	Advanced	3	12–15
Pelvic Tilts	Beginner	1	8–10
	Intermediate	2	10–12
	Advanced	3	10–15

Stretch

EXERCISE	SETS	HOLD
Hamstring Stretch: Single Leg Knee to Chest	3	15–60 Seconds
Hyper-Arch on Exercise Ball	3	15–60 Seconds
One Leg Forward Flexion	3	15–60 Seconds

INCREASE STRENGTH: WEEK FIVE / DAY 7

Aerobic

EXERCISE OPTIONS:	TIME:
Walking/Treadmill/Swimming/Biking/ Elliptical, Stairmaster/Aerobic	7 Minutes Heart Rate Goal: Between 65%–75%

Strength Training: Lower Body

CHOOSE TWO EXERCISES FOR EACH BODY PART:

SETS AND REPS:

Beginner:
Sets: 1
Reps: 8–10

Intermediate:
Sets: 2
Reps: 10–12

Advanced:
Sets: 3
Reps: 12–15

Glutes and Hips
- Plié Squats
- Dumbbell Squats
- Squats on Smith Machine
- Reverse Lunges*

Front of Legs
- Leg Extensions Using Ankle Weights
- Seated Leg Extension
- Inner Thigh Squats (Froggies)*
- Lying Bent Knee Leg Lifts*

Back of Legs
- Standing Hamstring Curls Using Ankle Weights

- Hamstring Curls Using Ankle Weights Over Bench, Chair or Ball
- Machine Hamstring Curls
- Standing Hamstring Curls*

Calves
- Standing Heel Raises Using Dumbbells
- Machine Heel Raises
- Heel Raises*

*Equipment-Free Exercise

Core

EXERCISE	FITNESS LEVEL	SETS	REPS
Quadruped Using Ankle Weights	Beginner	1	8–10
	Intermediate	2	10–12
	Advanced	3	10–15
Crunches on Exercise Bench Using Resistance Ball	Beginner	1	8–10
	Intermediate	2	10–12
	Advanced	3	12–15
Pelvic Tilts	Beginner	1	8–10
	Intermediate	2	10–12
	Advanced	3	10–15

Stretch

EXERCISE	SETS	HOLD
Hamstring Stretch: Single Leg Knee to Chest	3	15–60 Seconds
Quadriceps Stretch: Side-Lying Bent-Leg Stretch	3	15–60 Seconds
Hyper-Arch on Exercise Ball	3	15–60 Seconds

INCREASE STRENGTH: WEEK SIX / DAY 1

Aerobic

EXERCISE OPTIONS:	TIME:
Walking/Treadmill/Swimming/Biking/ Elliptical, Stairmaster/Aerobic	10 Minutes Heart Rate Goal: Between 65%–75%

Strength Training: Upper Body

CHOOSE TWO EXERCISES FOR EACH BODY PART:

SETS AND REPS:

Beginner:
Sets: 1
Reps: 8–10

Intermediate:
Sets: 2
Reps: 10–12

Advanced:
Sets: 3
Reps 12–15

Chest
- Flyes on Pec Machine
- Chest Press on Bench Using Body Bar or Smith Machine
- Dumbbell Presses Over Exercise Ball
- Presses*

Back
- Lat Pull-Downs
- Seated Low Rows
- Bent-Over Body Bar Rows
- Arm Pull-Downs

Biceps
- Biceps Curls Using Dumbbells
- Body Bar Biceps Curls

- Cable Biceps Curls
- Isometric Biceps Curls*

Triceps
- Triceps Extensions Pull-Downs
- One-Arm Overhead Triceps Extension
- Lying Triceps Extension
- Overhead Triceps Extension*

Shoulders
- One Arm Front Delt Lifts Using Dumbbells
- Shoulder Press Machine
- Reverse Flyes on Ball Using Dumbbells
- Overhead Presses

*Equipment-Free Exercises

Core

EXERCISE	FITNESS LEVEL	SETS	REPS
Classic Crunches*	Beginner	1	8–10
	Intermediate	2	10–12
	Advanced	3	10–15
Cycle Rotations	Beginner	1	8–10
	Intermediate	2	10–12
	Advanced	3	12–15
Quadruped Using Ankle Weights	Beginner	1	8–10
	Intermediate	2	10–12
	Advanced	3	10–15

Stretch

EXERCISE	SETS	HOLD
Hamstring Stretch: Single Leg Knee to Chest	3	15–60 Seconds
Hyper-Arch on Exercise Ball	3	15–60 Seconds
Biceps/Triceps Stretches	3	15–60 Seconds

INCREASE STRENGTH: WEEK SIX/ DAY 2

Aerobic

EXERCISE OPTIONS:	TIME:
Walking/Treadmill/Swimming/Biking/ Elliptical, Stairmaster/Aerobic Video	30 Minutes Heart Rate Goal: Between 65%–75%

Core

EXERCISE	FITNESS LEVEL	SETS	REPS
Back Extensions on Exercise Ball	Beginner	1	8–10
	Intermediate	2	10–12
	Advanced	3	10–15
Kegels	Beginner	1	8–10
	Intermediate	2	10–12
	Advanced	3	12–15
Ball Crunches	Beginner	1	8–10
	Intermediate	2	10–12
	Advanced	3	10–15

Stretch

EXERCISE	SETS	HOLD
Spinal Twist	3	15–60 Seconds
Hyper-Arch on Exercise Ball	3	15–60 Seconds
Piriformis Stretch	3	15–60 Seconds

INCREASE STRENGTH: WEEK SIX/ DAY 3

Aerobic

EXERCISE OPTIONS:	TIME:
Walking/Treadmill/Swimming/Biking/ Elliptical, Stairmaster/Aerobic	10 Minutes Heart Rate Goal: Between 65%–75%

Strength Training: Lower Body

CHOOSE ONE EXERCISE FOR EACH BODY PART:

SETS AND REPS:

Beginner:
Sets: 1
Reps: 8–10

Intermediate:
Sets: 2
Reps: 10–12

Advanced:
Sets: 3
Reps 12–15

Glutes and Hips
- Side-Lying Leg Lifts Using Exercise Band
- Step-Ups Using Barbell or Dumbbells
- Single Leg Lunges Using Resistance Ball
- Stationary Lunges*

Front of Legs
- Leg Extensions Using Ankle Weights
- Seated Leg Extension
- Inner Thigh Ball Squeezes
- Lying Bent Knee Leg Lifts*

Back of Legs
- Standing Hamstring Curls Using Ankle Weights
- Hamstring Curls Using Ankle Weights Over Bench, Chair or Ball
- Machine Hamstring Curls
- Standing Hamstring Curls*

Calves
- Standing Heel Raises Using Dumbbells
- Machine Heel Raises
- Heel Raises*

*Equipment-Free Exercise

Core

EXERCISE	FITNESS LEVEL	SETS	REPS
Quadruped Using Ankle Weights	Beginner	1	8–10
	Intermediate	2	10–12
	Advanced	3	10–15
Crunches on Exercise Bench Using Resistance Ball	Beginner	1	8–10
	Intermediate	2	10–12
	Advanced	3	12–15
Pelvic Tilts	Beginner	1	8–10
	Intermediate	2	10–12
	Advanced	3	10–15

Stretch

EXERCISE	SETS	HOLD
One-Leg Forward Flexion	3	15–60 Seconds
Quadriceps Stretch: Side-Lying Bent-Leg Stretch	3	15–60 Seconds
Hyper-Arch on Exercise Ball	3	15–60 Seconds

INCREASE STRENGTH: WEEK SIX/ DAY 4

Aerobic

EXERCISE OPTIONS:	TIME:
Walking/Treadmill/Swimming/Biking/ Elliptical, Stairmaster/Aerobic Video	30 Minutes Heart Rate Goal: Between 65%–75%

Core

EXERCISE	FITNESS LEVEL	SETS	REPS
Isometric Squeezes	Beginner	1	8–10
	Intermediate	2	10–12
	Advanced	3	10–15
Kegels	Beginner	1	8–10
	Intermediate	2	10–12
	Advanced	3	12–15
Plank or Modified Plank	Beginner	1	8–10
	Intermediate	2	10–12
	Advanced	3	10–15

Stretch

EXERCISE	SETS	HOLD
Hamstring Stretch: Single Leg Knee to Chest	3	15–60 Seconds
Spinal Twist	3	15–60 Seconds
Piriformis Stretch	3	15–60 Seconds

INCREASE STRENGTH: WEEK SIX/ DAY 5

Aerobic

EXERCISE OPTIONS:	TIME:
Walking/Treadmill/Swimming/Biking/ Elliptical, Stairmaster/Aerobic	10 Minutes Heart Rate Goal: Between 65%–75%

Strength Training: Upper Body

CHOOSE ONE EXERCISE FOR EACH BODY PART:

SETS AND REPS:

Beginner:
Sets: 1
Reps: 8–10

Intermediate:
Sets: 2
Reps: 10–12

Advanced:
Sets: 3
Reps 12–15

Chest
- Flyes on Pec Machine
- Chest Press on Bench Using Body Bar or Smith Machine
- Dumbbell Presses Over Exercise Ball
- Presses*

Back
- Lat Pull-Downs
- Seated Low Rows
- Bent-Over Body Bar Rows
- Arm Pull-Downs

Biceps
- Biceps Curls Using Dumbbells
- Body Bar Biceps Curls

- Cable Biceps Curls
- Isometric Biceps Curls*

Triceps
- Triceps Extensions Pull-Downs
- One-Arm Overhead Triceps Extension
- Lying Triceps Extension
- Overhead Triceps Extension*

Shoulders
- One Arm Front Delt Lifts Using Dumbbells
- Shoulder Press Machine
- Reverse Flyes on Ball Using Dumbbells
- Overhead Presses

*Equipment-Free Exercises

Core

EXERCISE	FITNESS LEVEL	SETS	REPS
Classic Crunches*	Beginner	1	8–10
	Intermediate	2	10–12
	Advanced	3	10–15
Cycle Rotations	Beginner	1	8–10
	Intermediate	2	10–12
	Advanced	3	12–15
Quadruped Using Ankle Weights	Beginner	1	8–10
	Intermediate	2	10–12
	Advanced	3	10–15

─────────────── *Stretch* ───────────────

EXERCISE	SETS	HOLD
Hamstring Stretch: Single Leg Knee to Chest	3	15–60 Seconds
Hyper-Arch on Exercise Ball	3	15–60 Seconds
Biceps/Triceps Stretches	3	15–60 Seconds

INCREASE STRENGTH: WEEK SIX/ DAY 6
OPTIONAL: REST DAY

─────────────── *Aerobic* ───────────────

EXERCISE OPTIONS:	TIME:
Walking/Treadmill/Swimming/Biking/ Elliptical, Stairmaster/Aerobic Video	30 Minutes Heart Rate Goal: Between 65%–75%

─────────────── *Core* ───────────────

EXERCISE	FITNESS LEVEL	SETS	REPS
Back Extensions on Exercise Ball	Beginner	1	8–10
	Intermediate	2	10–12
	Advanced	3	10–15
Kegels	Beginner	1	8–10
	Intermediate	2	10–12
	Advanced	3	12–15
Ball Crunches	Beginner	1	8–10
	Intermediate	2	10–12
	Advanced	3	10–15

Stretch

EXERCISE	SETS	HOLD
Spinal Twist	3	15–60 Seconds
Hyper-Arch on Exercise Ball	3	15–60 Seconds
Piriformis Stretch	3	15–60 Seconds

INCREASE STRENGTH: WEEK SIX/ DAY 7

Aerobic

EXERCISE OPTIONS:	TIME:
Walking/Treadmill/Swimming/Biking/ Elliptical, Stairmaster/Aerobic	10 Minutes Heart Rate Goal: Between 65%–75%

Strength Training: Lower Body

CHOOSE TWO EXERCISES FOR EACH BODY PART

SETS AND REPS:

Beginner:
Sets: 1
Reps: 8–10

Intermediate:
Sets: 2
Reps: 10–12

Advanced:
Sets: 3
Reps 12–15

Glutes and Hips
- Side-Lying Leg Lifts Using Exercise Band
- Step-Ups Using Barbell or Dumbbells
- Single Leg Lunges Using Resistance Ball
- Stationary Lunges*

Front of Legs
- Leg Extensions Using Ankle Weights
- Seated Leg Extension
- Inner Thigh Ball Squeezes
- Lying Bent Knee Leg Lifts*

Back of Legs
- Standing Hamstring Curls Using Ankle Weights

- Hamstring Curls Using Ankle Weights Over Bench, Chair or Ball
- Machine Hamstring Curls
- Standing Hamstring Curls*

Calves
- Standing Heel Raises Using Dumbbells
- Machine Heel Raises
- Heel Raises*

*Equipment-Free Exercise

────────────────────── *Core* ──────────────────────

EXERCISE	FITNESS LEVEL	SETS	REPS
Quadruped Using Ankle Weights	Beginner	1	8–10
	Intermediate	2	10–12
	Advanced	3	10–15
Crunches on Exercise Bench Using Resistance Ball	Beginner	1	8–10
	Intermediate	2	10–12
	Advanced	3	12–15
Pelvic Tilts	Beginner	1	8–10
	Intermediate	2	10–12
	Advanced	3	10–15

────────────────────── *Stretch* ──────────────────────

EXERCISE	SETS	HOLD
One-Leg Forward Flexion	3	15–60 Seconds
Quadriceps Stretch: Side-Lying Bent-Leg Stretch	3	15–60 Seconds
Hyper-Arch on Exercise Ball	3	15–60 Seconds

Anti-Aging Workout System 3
Goal: Cardiovascular Health, Tone, and Firm

CARDIOVASCULAR HEALTH: WEEK ONE/ DAY 1

Aerobic

EXERCISE OPTIONS:	TIME:
Walking/Treadmill/Swimming/Biking/ Elliptical, Stairmaster/Aerobic Video	25 Minutes Heart Rate Goal: Between 70%–80%

Core

EXERCISE	FITNESS LEVEL	SETS	REPS
Classic Crunches	Beginner	1	8–10
	Intermediate	2	10–12
	Advanced	3	10–15
Cycle Rotations	Beginner	1	8–10
	Intermediate	2	10–12
	Advanced	3	12–15
Reverse Leg Lifts Using Ankle Weights	Beginner	1	8–10
	Intermediate	2	10–12
	Advanced	3	10–15

Stretch

EXERCISE	SETS	HOLD
Hamstring Stretch: Single Leg Knee to Chest	3	15–60 Seconds
Piriformis Stretch	3	15–60 Seconds
Spinal Twist	3	15–60 Seconds

CARDIOVASCULAR HEALTH: WEEK ONE/ DAY 2

Aerobic

EXERCISE OPTIONS:	TIME:
Walking/Treadmill/Swimming/Biking/ Elliptical, Stairmaster/Aerobic Video	25 Minutes Heart Rate Goal: Between 70–80%

Core

EXERCISE	FITNESS LEVEL	SETS	REPS
Reverse Leg Lifts with Ankle Weights	Beginner	1	8–10
	Intermediate	2	10–12
	Advanced	3	10–15
Cycle Rotations	Beginner	1	8–10
	Intermediate	2	10–12
	Advanced	3	12–15
Back Extensions on Exercise Ball	Beginner	1	8–10
	Intermediate	2	10–12
	Advanced	3	10–15

Stretch

EXERCISE	SETS	HOLD
One Leg Forward Flexion	3	15–60 Seconds
Hyper-Arch on Exercise Ball	3	15–60 Seconds
Spinal Twist	3	15–60 Seconds

CARDIOVASCULAR HEALTH: WEEK ONE/ DAY 3

Aerobic

EXERCISE OPTIONS:	TIME:
Walking/Treadmill/Swimming/Biking/ Elliptical, Stairmaster/Aerobic	15 Minutes Heart Rate Goal: Between 70–80%

Strength Training: Lower and Upper Body

CHOOSE ONE EXERCISE FOR EACH BODY PART:

SETS AND REPS:

Beginner:
Sets: 1
Reps: 8–10

Intermediate:
Sets: 2
Reps: 10–12

Advanced:
Sets: 3
Reps: 12–15

Front of Legs
• Plié Squats Against Ball
• Seated Leg Extension
• Leg Extensions Using Ankle Weights
• Lying Bent Knee Leg Lifts*

Back of Legs
• Standing Hamstring Curls Using Ankle Weights
• Hamstring Curls Using Ankle Weights Over Bench, Chair or Ball
• Machine Hamstring Curls
• Standing Hamstring Curls*

Chest
• Chest Flyes Using Dumbbells on Flat Bench

• Chest Press on Bench Using Body Bar or Smith Machine
• Dumbbell Presses Over Exercise Ball
• Floor Push-Ups*

Back
• Lat Pull-Downs
• One-Arm Kneeling Rows
• Bent-Over Body Bar Rows
• Arm Pull-Downs*

*Equipment-Free Exercise

Core

EXERCISE	FITNESS LEVEL	SETS	REPS
Plank or Modified Plank	Beginner	1	8–10
	Intermediate	2	10–12
	Advanced	3	10–15
Ball Crunches	Beginner	1	8–10
	Intermediate	2	10–12
	Advanced	3	12–15
Kegels	Beginner	1	8–10
	Intermediate	2	10–12
	Advanced	3	10–15

―――――――― *Stretch* ――――――――

EXERCISE	SETS	HOLD
Hamstring Stretch: Single Leg Knee to Chest	3	15–60 Seconds
Quadriceps Stretch: Side-Lying Bent-Leg Stretch	3	15–60 Seconds
Hyper-Arch on Exercise Ball	3	15–60 Seconds

CARDIOVASCULAR HEALTH: WEEK ONE/ DAY 4

―――――――― *Aerobic* ――――――――

EXERCISE OPTIONS:	TIME:
Walking/Treadmill/Swimming/Biking/ Elliptical, Stairmaster/Aerobic Video	25 Minutes Heart Rate Goal: Between 70–80%

―――――――― *Core* ――――――――

EXERCISE	FITNESS LEVEL	SETS	REPS
Isometric Squeezes	Beginner	1	8–10
	Intermediate	2	10–12
	Advanced	3	10–15
Pelvic Tilts	Beginner	1	8–10
	Intermediate	2	10–12
	Advanced	3	12–15
Crunches on Flat Bench Using Resistance Ball	Beginner	1	8–10
	Intermediate	2	10–12
	Advanced	3	10–15

―――――――― *Stretch* ――――――――

EXERCISE	SETS	HOLD
Spinal Twist	3	15–60 Seconds
Hyper-Arch on Exercise Ball	3	15–60 Seconds
Piriformis Stretch	3	15–60 Seconds

CARDIOVASCULAR HEALTH: WEEK ONE/ DAY 5

Aerobic

EXERCISE OPTIONS:	TIME:
Walking/Treadmill/Swimming/Biking/ Elliptical, Stairmaster/Aerobic	15 Minutes Heart Rate Goal: Between 70–80%

Strength Training: Lower and Upper Body

CHOOSE ONE EXERCISE FOR EACH BODY PART:

SETS AND REPS:

Beginner:
Sets: 1
Reps: 8–10

Intermediate:
Sets: 2
Reps: 10–12

Advanced:
Sets: 3
Reps: 12–15

Glutes and Hips
- Ball Squats
- Side-Lying Leg Lifts Using Exercise Band
- Reverse Lunges Using Ankle Weights
- Sit Downs*

Calves
- Standing Heel Raises Using Dumbbells
- Machine Heel Raises
- Heel Raises*

Biceps
- Biceps Curls Using Dumbbells
- Seated One-Arm Biceps Curls

- Cable Biceps Curls
- Isometric Biceps Curls*

Triceps
- Triceps Extension Pull-Downs
- One-Arm Overhead Triceps Extension
- Lying Triceps Extension
- Triceps Wall Push-Ups*

Shoulders
- Angled One-Arm Side Raises
- Overhead Presses Using Dumbbells
- Reverse Flyes on Ball Using Dumbbells
- Reverse Flyes*

*Equipment-Free Exercise

Core

EXERCISE	FITNESS LEVEL	SETS	REPS
Back Extensions on Exercise Ball	Beginner	1	8–10
	Intermediate	2	10–12
	Advanced	3	10–15
Cycle Rotations	Beginner	1	8–10
	Intermediate	2	10–12
	Advanced	3	12–15
Sitting Leg Lifts	Beginner	1	8–10
	Intermediate	2	10–12
	Advanced	3	10–15

Stretch

EXERCISE	SETS	HOLD
One Leg Forward Flexion	3	15–60 Seconds
Piriformis Stretch	3	15–60 Seconds
Spinal Twist	3	15–60 Seconds

CARDIOVASCULAR HEALTH: WEEK ONE/ DAY 6

Aerobic

EXERCISE OPTIONS:	TIME:
Walking/Treadmill/Swimming/Biking/ Elliptical, Stairmaster/Aerobic Video	25 Minutes Heart Rate Goal: Between 70–80%

Core

EXERCISE	FITNESS LEVEL	SETS	REPS
Classic Crunches	Beginner	1	8–10
	Intermediate	2	10–12
	Advanced	3	10–15
Cycle Rotations	Beginner	1	8–10
	Intermediate	2	10–12
	Advanced	3	12–15
Reverse Leg Lifts Using Ankle Weights	Beginner	1	8–10
	Intermediate	2	10–12
	Advanced	3	10–15

Stretch

EXERCISE	SETS	HOLD
Hamstring Stretch: Single Leg Knee to Chest	3	15–60 Seconds
Piriformis Stretch	3	15–60 Seconds
Spinal Twist	3	15–60 Seconds

CARDIOVASCULAR HEALTH: WEEK ONE/ DAY 7
OPTIONAL: REST DAY

Aerobic

EXERCISE OPTIONS:	TIME:
Walking/Treadmill/Swimming/Biking/ Elliptical, Stairmaster/Aerobic Video	15 Minutes Heart Rate Goal: Between 70–80%

Core

EXERCISE	FITNESS LEVEL	SETS	REPS
Leg Lifts	Beginner	1	8–10
	Intermediate	2	10–12
	Advanced	3	10–15
Kegels	Beginner	1	8–10
	Intermediate	2	10–12
	Advanced	3	12–15
Pelvic Tilts	Beginner	1	8–10
	Intermediate	2	10–12
	Advanced	3	10–15

Stretch

EXERCISE	SETS	HOLD
Hamstring Stretch: Single Leg Knee to Chest	3	15–60 Seconds
Hyper-Arch on Exercise Ball	3	15–60 Seconds
One Leg Forward Flexion	3	15–60 Seconds

CARDIOVASCULAR HEALTH: WEEK TWO/ DAY 1

Aerobic

EXERCISE OPTIONS:	TIME:
Walking/Treadmill/Swimming/Biking/ Elliptical, Stairmaster/Aerobic Video	25 Minutes Heart Rate Goal: Between 70–80%

Core

EXERCISE	FITNESS LEVEL	SETS	REPS
Ball Crunches	Beginner	1	8–10
	Intermediate	2	10–12
	Advanced	3	10–15
Lateral Side Drops on Ball	Beginner	1	8–10
	Intermediate	2	10–12
	Advanced	3	12–15
Reverse Leg Lifts with Ankle Weights	Beginner	1	8–10
	Intermediate	2	10–12
	Advanced	3	10–15

Stretch

EXERCISE	SETS	HOLD
Hamstring Stretch: Single Leg Knee to Chest	3	15–60 Seconds
Piriformis Stretch	3	15–60 Seconds
Spinal Twist	3	15–60 Seconds

CARDIOVASCULAR HEALTH: WEEK TWO/ DAY 2

Aerobic

EXERCISE OPTIONS:	TIME:
Walking/Treadmill/Swimming/Biking/ Elliptical, Stairmaster/Aerobic Video	25 Minutes Heart Rate Goal: Between 70–80%

Core

EXERCISE	FITNESS LEVEL	SETS	REPS
Reverse Leg Lifts Using Ankle Weights	Beginner	1	8–10
	Intermediate	2	10–12
	Advanced	3	10–15
Plank or Modified Plank	Beginner	1	8–10
	Intermediate	2	10–12
	Advanced	3	12–15
Lateral Drops on Exercise Ball	Beginner	1	8–10
	Intermediate	2	10–12
	Advanced	3	10–15

Stretch

EXERCISE	SETS	HOLD
One Leg Forward Flexion	3	15–60 Seconds
Piriformis Stretch	3	15–60 Seconds
Spinal Twist	3	15–60 Seconds

CARDIOVASCULAR HEALTH: WEEK TWO/ DAY 3

───── *Aerobic* ─────

EXERCISE OPTIONS:	TIME:
Walking/Treadmill/Swimming/Biking/ Elliptical, Stairmaster/Aerobic	15 Minutes Heart Rate Goal: Between 70–80%

───── *Strength Training: Lower and Upper Body* ─────

CHOOSE ONE EXERCISE FOR EACH BODY PART:

SETS AND REPS:

Beginner:
Sets: 1
Reps: 8–10

Intermediate:
Sets: 2
Reps: 10–12

Advanced:
Sets: 3
Reps 12–15

Glutes and Hips
- Ball Squats
- Step-Ups Using Barbell or Dumbbells
- Squats on Smith Machine
- Reverse Lunges*

Calves
- Standing Heel Raises Using Dumbbells
- Machine Heel Raises
- Heel Raises*

Biceps
- Biceps Curls Using Dumbbells
- Body Bar Biceps Curls
- Cable Biceps Curls
- Isometric Biceps Curls*

Triceps
- Triceps Extensions Pull-Downs
- One-Arm Overhead Triceps Extension
- Lying Triceps Extension
- Overhead Triceps Extension*

Shoulders
- One Arm Front Delt Lifts Using Dumbbells
- Shoulder Press Machine
- Reverse Flyes on Ball Using Dumbbells
- Overhead Presses

*Equipment-Free Exercises

───── *Core* ─────

EXERCISE	FITNESS LEVEL	SETS	REPS
Leg Lifts	Beginner	1	8–10
	Intermediate	2	10–12
	Advanced	3	10–15
Crunches on Exercise Bench Using Resistance Ball	Beginner	1	8–10
	Intermediate	2	10–12
	Advanced	3	12–15
Pelvic Tilts	Beginner	1	8–10
	Intermediate	2	10–12
	Advanced	3	10–15

Stretch

EXERCISE	SETS	HOLD
One Leg Forward Flexion	3	15–60 Seconds
Quadriceps Stretch: Side-Lying Bent-Leg Stretch	3	15–60 Seconds
Hyper-Arch on Exercise Ball	3	15–60 Seconds

CARDIOVASCULAR HEALTH: WEEK TWO/ DAY 4

Aerobic

EXERCISE OPTIONS:	TIME:
Walking/Treadmill/Swimming/Biking/ Elliptical, Stairmaster/Aerobic Video	25 Minutes Heart Rate Goal: Between 65%–75%

Core

EXERCISE	FITNESS LEVEL	SETS	REPS
Back Extensions on Exercise Ball	Beginner	1	8–10
	Intermediate	2	10–12
	Advanced	3	10–15
Kegels	Beginner	1	8–10
	Intermediate	2	10–12
	Advanced	3	12–15
Ball Crunches	Beginner	1	8–10
	Intermediate	2	10–12
	Advanced	3	10–15

Stretch

EXERCISE	SETS	HOLD
Spinal Twist	3	15–60 Seconds
Hyper-Arch on Exercise Ball	3	15–60 Seconds
Piriformis Stretch	3	15–60 Seconds

CARDIOVASCULAR HEALTH: WEEK TWO/ DAY 5

Aerobic

EXERCISE OPTIONS:	TIME:
Walking/Treadmill/Swimming/Biking/ Elliptical, Stairmaster/Aerobic	15 Minutes Heart Rate Goal: Between 70–80%

Strength Training: Lower and Upper Body

CHOOSE ONE EXERCISE FOR EACH BODY PART:

SETS AND REPS:

Beginner:
Sets: 1
Reps: 8–10

Intermediate:
Sets: 2
Reps: 10–12

Advanced:
Sets: 3
Reps 12–15

Front of Legs
- Leg Extensions Using Ankle Weights
- Seated Leg Extension
- Side-Lying Inner Thigh Lifts Using Ankle Weights
- Lying Bent Knee Leg Lifts*

Back of Legs
- Standing Hamstring Curls Using Ankle Weights
- Hamstring Curls Using Ankle Weights Over Bench, Chair or Ball
- Machine Hamstring Curls
- Standing Hamstring Curls*

Chest
- Flyes on Pec Machine
- Chest Press on Bench Using Body Bar or Smith Machine
- Dumbbell Presses Over Exercise Ball
- Presses*

Back
- Lat Pull-Downs
- Seated Low Rows
- Bent-Over Body Bar Rows
- Arm Pull-Downs

*Equipment-Free Exercises

Core

EXERCISE	FITNESS LEVEL	SETS	REPS
Classic Crunches*	Beginner	1	8–10
	Intermediate	2	10–12
	Advanced	3	10–15
Cycle Rotations	Beginner	1	8–10
	Intermediate	2	10–12
	Advanced	3	12–15
Quadruped Using Ankle Weights	Beginner	1	8–10
	Intermediate	2	10–12
	Advanced	3	10–15

Stretch

EXERCISE	SETS	HOLD
Hamstring Stretch: Single Leg Knee to Chest	3	15–60 Seconds
Hyper-Arch on Exercise Ball	3	15–60 Seconds
Biceps/Triceps Stretches	3	15–60 Seconds

CARDIOVASCULAR HEALTH: WEEK TWO/ DAY 6

Aerobic

EXERCISE OPTIONS:	TIME:
Walking/Treadmill/Swimming/Biking/ Elliptical, Stairmaster/Aerobic Video	25 Minutes Heart Rate Goal: Between 70–80%

Core

Exercise	Fitness Level	Sets	Reps
Isometric Squeezes	Beginner	1	8–10
	Intermediate	2	10–12
	Advanced	3	10–15
Kegels	Beginner	1	8–10
	Intermediate	2	10–12
	Advanced	3	12–15
Plank or Modified Plank	Beginner	1	8–10
	Intermediate	2	10–12
	Advanced	3	10–15

Stretch

EXERCISE	SETS	HOLD
Hamstring Stretch: Single Leg Knee to Chest	3	15–60 Seconds
Spinal Twist	3	15–60 Seconds
Piriformis Stretch	3	15–60 Seconds

CARDIOVASCULAR HEALTH: WEEK TWO/ DAY 7
OPTIONAL: REST DAY

Aerobic

EXERCISE OPTIONS:	TIME:
Walking/Treadmill/Swimming/Biking/ Elliptical, Stairmaster/Aerobic Video	15 Minutes Heart Rate Goal: Between 70–80%

Core

EXERCISE	FITNESS LEVEL	SETS	REPS
Ball Crunches	Beginner	1	8–10
	Intermediate	2	10–12
	Advanced	3	10–15
Lateral Side Drops on Ball	Beginner	1	8–10
	Intermediate	2	10–12
	Advanced	3	12–15
Reverse Leg Lifts with Ankle Weights	Beginner	1	8–10
	Intermediate	2	10–12
	Advanced	3	10–15

Stretch

EXERCISE	SETS	HOLD
Hamstring Stretch: Single Leg Knee to Chest	3	15–60 Seconds
Piriformis Stretch	3	15–60 Seconds
Spinal Twist	3	15–60 Seconds

CARDIOVASCULAR HEALTH: WEEK THREE/ DAY 1

Aerobic

EXERCISE OPTIONS:	TIME:
Walking/Treadmill/Swimming/Biking/ Elliptical, Stairmaster/Aerobic Video	30 Minutes Heart Rate Goal: Between 70–85%

Core

EXERCISE	FITNESS LEVEL	SETS	REPS
Classic Crunches*	Beginner	1	8–10
	Intermediate	2	10–12
	Advanced	3	10–15
Cycle Rotations*	Beginner	1	8–10
	Intermediate	2	10–12
	Advanced	3	12–15
Reverse Leg Lifts Using Ankle Weights	Beginner	1	8–10
	Intermediate	2	10–12
	Advanced	3	10–15

Stretch

EXERCISE	SETS	HOLD
One Leg Forward Flexion	3	15–60 Seconds
Piriformis Stretch	3	15–60 Seconds
Spinal Twist	3	15–60 Seconds

CARDIOVASCULAR HEALTH: WEEK THREE/ DAY 2

Aerobic

EXERCISE OPTIONS:	TIME:
Walking/Treadmill/Swimming/Biking/ Elliptical, Stairmaster/Aerobic Video	30 Minutes Heart Rate Goal: Between 70–85%

Core

EXERCISE	FITNESS LEVEL	SETS	REPS
Reverse Leg Lifts with Ankle Weights	Beginner	1	8–10
	Intermediate	2	10–12
	Advanced	3	10–15
Cycle Rotations	Beginner	1	8–10
	Intermediate	2	10–12
	Advanced	3	12–15
Back Extensions on Exercise Ball	Beginner	1	8–10
	Intermediate	2	10–12
	Advanced	3	10–15

Stretch

EXERCISE	SETS	HOLD
One Leg Forward Flexion	3	15–60 Seconds
Hyper-Arch on Exercise Ball	3	15–60 Seconds
Spinal Twist	3	15–60 Seconds

CARDIOVASCULAR HEALTH: WEEK THREE/ DAY 3

Aerobic

EXERCISE OPTIONS:	TIME:
Walking/Treadmill/Swimming/Biking/ Elliptical, Stairmaster/Aerobic	15 Minutes Heart Rate Goal: Between 65%–75%

Strength Training: Lower and Upper Body

CHOOSE ONE EXERCISE FOR EACH BODY PART:

SETS AND REPS:

Beginner:
Sets: 1
Reps: 8–10

Intermediate:
Sets: 2
Reps: 10–12

Advanced:
Sets: 3
Reps 12–15

Front of Legs
• Plié Squats Against Ball
• Seated Leg Extension
• Leg Extensions Using Ankle Weights
• Lying Bent Knee Leg Lifts*

Back of Legs
• Standing Hamstring Curls Using Ankle Weights
• Hamstring Curls Using Ankle Weights Over Bench, Chair or Ball
• Machine Hamstring Curls
• Standing Hamstring Curls*

Chest
• Ball Push-Ups

• Chest Press Using Body Bar/Smith Machine
• Dumbbell Presses on Ball
• Wall Push-Ups*

Back
• Lat Pull Downs
• One-Arm Kneeling Rows
• Machine Assisted Pull-Ups
• Back Rows*

*Equipment-Free Exercises

Core

EXERCISE	FITNESS LEVEL	SETS	REPS
Ball Crunches	Beginner	1	8–10
	Intermediate	2	10–12
	Advanced	3	10–15
Lateral Side Drops on Ball	Beginner	1	8–10
	Intermediate	2	10–12
	Advanced	3	12–15
Sitting Leg Lifts	Beginner	1	8–10
	Intermediate	2	10–12
	Advanced	3	10–15

Stretch

EXERCISE	SETS	HOLD
Hamstring Stretch: Single Leg Knee to Chest	3	15–60 Seconds
Piriformis Stretch	3	15–60 Seconds
Biceps/Triceps Stretches	3	15–60 Seconds

CARDIOVASCULAR HEALTH: WEEK THREE/ DAY 4

Aerobic

EXERCISE OPTIONS:	TIME:
Walking/Treadmill/Swimming/Biking/ Elliptical, Stairmaster/Aerobic Video	30 Minutes Heart Rate Goal: Between 70–85%

Core

EXERCISE	FITNESS LEVEL	SETS	REPS
Isometric Squeezes	Beginner	1	8–10
	Intermediate	2	10–12
	Advanced	3	10–15
Pelvic Tilts	Beginner	1	8–10
	Intermediate	2	10–12
	Advanced	3	12–15
Crunches on Flat Bench Using Resistance Ball	Beginner	1	8–10
	Intermediate	2	10–12
	Advanced	3	10–15

Stretch

EXERCISE	SETS	HOLD
Spinal Twist	3	15–60 Seconds
One Leg Forward Flexion	3	15–60 Seconds
Hyper-Arch on Exercise Ball	3	15–60 Seconds

CARDIOVASCULAR HEALTH: WEEK THREE/ DAY 5

Aerobic

EXERCISE OPTIONS:	TIME:
Walking/Treadmill/Swimming/Biking/ Elliptical, Stairmaster/Aerobic	15 Minutes Heart Rate Goal: Between 65%–75%

Strength Training: Lower and Upper Body

CHOOSE ONE EXERCISE FOR EACH BODY PART:

SETS AND REPS:

Beginner:
Sets: 1
Reps: 8–10

Intermediate:
Sets: 2
Reps: 10–12

Advanced:
Sets: 3
Reps 12–15

Glutes and Hips
- Ball Squats
- Side-Lying Leg Lifts Using Exercise Band
- Reverse Lunges Using Ankle Weights
- Sit Downs*

Calves
- Standing Heel Raises Using Dumbbells
- Machine Heel Raises
- Heel Raises*

Biceps
- Biceps Curls Using Dumbbells
- Body Bar Biceps Curls
- Cable Biceps Curls
- Isometric Biceps Curls*

Triceps
- Triceps Extension Pull-Downs
- One-Arm Overhead Triceps Extension
- Lying Triceps Extension
- Triceps V-Backs*

Shoulders
- One Arm Front Delt Lifts Using Dumbbells
- Shoulder Press Machine
- Reverse Flyes on Ball Using Dumbbells
- Overhead Presses*

*Equipment-Free Exercise

Core

EXERCISE	FITNESS LEVEL	SETS	REPS
Plank or Modified Plank	Beginner	1	8–10
	Intermediate	2	10–12
	Advanced	3	10–15
Ball Crunches	Beginner	1	8–10
	Intermediate	2	10–12
	Advanced	3	12–15
Kegels	Beginner	1	8–10
	Intermediate	2	10–12
	Advanced	3	10–15

Stretch

EXERCISE	SETS	HOLD
Hamstring Stretch: Single Leg Knee to Chest	3	15–60 Seconds
Quadriceps Stretch: Side-Lying Bent-Leg Stretch	3	15–60 Seconds
Hyper-Arch on Exercise Ball	3	15–60 Seconds

CARDIOVASCULAR HEALTH: WEEK THREE/ DAY 6

Aerobic

EXERCISE OPTIONS:	TIME:
Walking/Treadmill/Swimming/Biking/ Elliptical, Stairmaster/Aerobic Video	30 Minutes Heart Rate Goal: Between 70–85%

Core

EXERCISE	FITNESS LEVEL	SETS	REPS
Isometric Squeezes	Beginner	1	8–10
	Intermediate	2	10–12
	Advanced	3	10–15
Kegels	Beginner	1	8–10
	Intermediate	2	10–12
	Advanced	3	12–15
Pelvic Tilts	Beginner	1	8–10
	Intermediate	2	10–12
	Advanced	3	10–15

Stretch

EXERCISE	SETS	HOLD
Hamstring Stretch: Single Leg Knee to Chest	3	15–60 Seconds
Hyper-Arch on Exercise Ball	3	15–60 Seconds
One Leg Forward Flexion	3	15–60 Seconds

CARDIOVASCULAR HEALTH: WEEK THREE/ DAY 7
OPTIONAL: REST DAY

────────────────── *Aerobic* ──────────────────

EXERCISE OPTIONS:	TIME:
Walking/Treadmill/Swimming/Biking/ Elliptical, Stairmaster/Aerobic Video	15 Minutes Heart Rate Goal: Between 70–85%

────────────────── *Core* ──────────────────

EXERCISE	FITNESS LEVEL	SETS	REPS
Classic Crunches*	Beginner	1	8–10
	Intermediate	2	10–12
	Advanced	3	10–15
Cycle Rotations*	Beginner	1	8–10
	Intermediate	2	10–12
	Advanced	3	12–15
Reverse Leg Lifts Using Ankle Weights	Beginner	1	8–10
	Intermediate	2	10–12
	Advanced	3	10–15

────────────────── *Stretch* ──────────────────

EXERCISE	SETS	HOLD
One Leg Forward Flexion	3	15–60 Seconds
Piriformis Stretch	3	15–60 Seconds
Spinal Twist	3	15–60 Seconds

CARDIOVASCULAR HEALTH: WEEK FOUR/ DAY 1

Aerobic

EXERCISE OPTIONS:	TIME:
Walking/Treadmill/Swimming/Biking/ Elliptical, Stairmaster/Aerobic Video	35 Minutes Heart Rate Goal: Between 70–85%

Core

EXERCISE	FITNESS LEVEL	SETS	REPS
Ball Crunches	Beginner	1	8–10
	Intermediate	2	10–12
	Advanced	3	10–15
Lateral Side Drops on Ball	Beginner	1	8–10
	Intermediate	2	10–12
	Advanced	3	12–15
Reverse Leg Lifts with Ankle Weights	Beginner	1	8–10
	Intermediate	2	10–12
	Advanced	3	10–15

Stretch

EXERCISE	SETS	HOLD
Hamstring Stretch: Single Leg Knee to Chest	3	15–60 Seconds
Piriformis Stretch	3	15–60 Seconds
Spinal Twist	3	15–60 Seconds

CARDIOVASCULAR HEALTH: WEEK FOUR/ DAY 2

Aerobic

EXERCISE OPTIONS:	TIME:
Walking/Treadmill/Swimming/Biking/ Elliptical, Stairmaster/Aerobic Video	35 Minutes Heart Rate Goal: Between 70–85%

Core

EXERCISE	FITNESS LEVEL	SETS	REPS
Isometric Squeezes	Beginner	1	8–10
	Intermediate	2	10–12
	Advanced	3	10–15
Kegels	Beginner	1	8–10
	Intermediate	2	10–12
	Advanced	3	12–15
Ball Crunches	Beginner	1	8–10
	Intermediate	2	10–12
	Advanced	3	10–15

Stretch

EXERCISE	SETS	HOLD
Spinal Twist	3	15–60 Seconds
Hyper-Arch on Exercise Ball	3	15–60 Seconds
Piriformis Stretch	3	15–60 Seconds

CARDIOVASCULAR HEALTH: WEEK FOUR/ DAY 3

Aerobic

EXERCISE OPTIONS:	TIME:
Walking/Treadmill/Swimming/Biking/ Elliptical, Stairmaster/Aerobic	15 Minutes Heart Rate Goal: Between 70–85%

Strength Training: Lower and Upper Body

CHOOSE ONE EXERCISE FOR EACH BODY PART:

SETS AND REPS:

Beginner:
Sets: 1
Reps: 8–10

Intermediate:
Sets: 2
Reps: 10–12

Advanced:
Sets: 3
Reps: 12–15

Front of Legs
- Leg Extensions Using Ankle Weights
- Seated Leg Extension
- Inner Thigh Squats (Froggies)*
- Lying Bent Knee Leg Lifts*

Back of Legs
- Standing Hamstring Curls Using Ankle Weights
- Hamstring Curls Using Ankle Weights Over Bench, Chair or Ball
- Machine Hamstring Curls
- Standing Hamstring Curls*

Chest
- Flyes on Pec Machine

- Chest Press on Bench Using Body Bar or Smith Machine
- Dumbbell Presses Over Exercise Ball
- Floor Push-Ups*

Back
- Lat Pull-Downs
- One-Arm Kneeling Rows
- Bent-Over Body Bar Rows
- Arm Pull-Downs*

*Equipment-Free Exercise

Core

EXERCISE	FITNESS LEVEL	SETS	REPS
Quadruped Using Ankle Weights	Beginner	1	8–10
	Intermediate	2	10–12
	Advanced	3	10–15
Crunches on Exercise Bench Using Resistance Ball	Beginner	1	8–10
	Intermediate	2	10–12
	Advanced	3	12–15
Pelvic Tilts	Beginner	1	8–10
	Intermediate	2	10–12
	Advanced	3	10–15

Stretch

EXERCISE	SETS	HOLD
Hamstring Stretch: Single Leg Knee to Chest	3	15–60 Seconds
Quadriceps Stretch: Side-Lying Bent-Leg Stretch	3	15–60 Seconds
Hyper-Arch on Exercise Ball	3	15–60 Seconds

CARDIOVASCULAR HEALTH: WEEK FOUR/ DAY 4

Aerobic

EXERCISE OPTIONS:	TIME:
Walking/Treadmill/Swimming/Biking/ Elliptical, Stairmaster/Aerobic Video	35 Minutes Heart Rate Goal: Between 70–85%

Core

EXERCISE	FITNESS LEVEL	SETS	REPS
Reverse Leg Lifts with Ankle Weights	Beginner	1	8–10
	Intermediate	2	10–12
	Advanced	3	10–15
Plank or Modified Plank	Beginner	1	8–10
	Intermediate	2	10–12
	Advanced	3	12–15
Lateral Drops on Exercise Ball	Beginner	1	8–10
	Intermediate	2	10–12
	Advanced	3	10–15

Stretch

EXERCISE	SETS	HOLD
One Leg Forward Flexion	3	15–60 Seconds
Piriformis Stretch	3	15–60 Seconds
Spinal Twist	3	15–60 Seconds

CARDIOVASCULAR HEALTH: WEEK FOUR/ DAY 5

Aerobic

EXERCISE OPTIONS:	TIME:
Walking/Treadmill/Swimming/Biking/ Elliptical, Stairmaster/Aerobic	15 Minutes Heart Rate Goal: Between 70–85%

Strength Training: Lower and Upper Body

CHOOSE ONE EXERCISE FOR EACH BODY PART:

SETS AND REPS:

Beginner:
Sets: 1
Reps: 8–10

Intermediate:
Sets: 2
Reps: 10–12

Advanced:
Sets: 3
Reps 12–15

Glutes and Hips
- Plié Squats
- Dumbbell Squats
- Squats on Smith Machine
- Reverse Lunges*

Calves
- Standing Heel Raises Using Dumbbells
- Machine Heel Raises
- Heel Raises*

Biceps
- Biceps Curls Using Dumbbells
- Seated One-Arm Biceps Curls
- Cable Biceps Curls
- Isometric Biceps Curls*

Triceps
- Triceps Extension Pull -Downs
- One-Arm Overhead Triceps Extension
- Lying Triceps Extension
- Triceps Wall Push-Ups*

Shoulders
- Angled One-Arm Side Raises
- Overhead Presses Using Dumbbells
- Reverse Flyes on Ball Using Dumbbells

*Equipment-Free Exercises

Core

EXERCISE	FITNESS LEVEL	SETS	REPS
Quadruped Using Ankle Weights	Beginner	1	8–10
	Intermediate	2	10–12
	Advanced	3	10–15
Crunches on Exercise Bench Using Resistance Ball	Beginner	1	8–10
	Intermediate	2	10–12
	Advanced	3	12–15
Pelvic Tilts	Beginner	1	8–10
	Intermediate	2	10–12
	Advanced	3	10–15

Stretch

EXERCISE	SETS	HOLD
Hamstring Stretch: Single Leg Knee to Chest	3	15–60 Seconds
Quadriceps Stretch: Side-Lying Bent-Leg Stretch	3	15–60 Seconds
Hyper-Arch on Exercise Ball	3	15–60 Seconds

CARDIOVASCULAR HEALTH: WEEK FOUR/ DAY 6

Aerobic

EXERCISE OPTIONS:	TIME:
Walking/Treadmill/Swimming/Biking/ Elliptical, Stairmaster/Aerobic Video	35 Minutes Heart Rate Goal: Between 70–85%

Core

EXERCISE	FITNESS LEVEL	SETS	REPS
Isometric Squeezes	Beginner	1	8–10
	Intermediate	2	10–12
	Advanced	3	10–15
Kegels	Beginner	1	8–10
	Intermediate	2	10–12
	Advanced	3	12–15
Plank or Modified Plank	Beginner	1	8–10
	Intermediate	2	10–12
	Advanced	3	10–15

Stretch

EXERCISE	SETS	HOLD
Hamstring Stretch: Single Leg Knee to Chest	3	15–60 Seconds
Spinal Twist	3	15–60 Seconds
Piriformis Stretch	3	15–60 Seconds

CARDIOVASCULAR HEALTH: WEEK FOUR/ DAY 7
OPTIONAL: REST DAY

Aerobic

EXERCISE OPTIONS:	TIME:
Walking/Treadmill/Swimming/Biking/ Elliptical, Stairmaster/Aerobic Video	15 Minutes Heart Rate Goal: Between 70–85%

Core

EXERCISE	FITNESS LEVEL	SETS	REPS
Ball Crunches	Beginner	1	8–10
	Intermediate	2	10–12
	Advanced	3	10–15
Lateral Side Drops on Ball	Beginner	1	8–10
	Intermediate	2	10–12
	Advanced	3	12–15
Reverse Leg Lifts with Ankle Weights	Beginner	1	8–10
	Intermediate	2	10–12
	Advanced	3	10–15

Stretch

EXERCISE	SETS	HOLD
Hamstring Stretch: Single Leg Knee to Chest	3	15–60 Seconds
Piriformis Stretch	3	15–60 Seconds
Spinal Twist	3	15–60 Seconds

CARDIOVASCULAR HEALTH: WEEK FIVE/ DAY 1

Aerobic

EXERCISE OPTIONS:	TIME:
Walking/Treadmill/Swimming/Biking/ Elliptical, Stairmaster/Aerobic Video	40 Minutes Heart Rate Goal: Between 70–85%

Core

EXERCISE	FITNESS LEVEL	SETS	REPS
Classic Crunches	Beginner	1	8–10
	Intermediate	2	10–12
	Advanced	3	10–15
Cycle Rotations	Beginner	1	8–10
	Intermediate	2	10–12
	Advanced	3	12–15
Reverse Leg Lifts Using Ankle Weights	Beginner	1	8–10
	Intermediate	2	10–12
	Advanced	3	10–15

Stretch

EXERCISE	SETS	HOLD
Hamstring Stretch: Single Leg Knee to Chest	3	15–60 Seconds
Piriformis Stretch	3	15–60 Seconds
Spinal Twist	3	15–60 Seconds

CARDIOVASCULAR HEALTH: WEEK FIVE/ DAY 2

Aerobic

EXERCISE OPTIONS:	TIME:
Walking/Treadmill/Swimming/Biking/ Elliptical, Stairmaster/Aerobic Video	40 Minutes Heart Rate Goal: Between 70–85%

Core

EXERCISE	FITNESS LEVEL	SETS	REPS
Reverse Leg Lifts with Ankle Weights	Beginner	1	8–10
	Intermediate	2	10–12
	Advanced	3	10–15
Cycle Rotations	Beginner	1	8–10
	Intermediate	2	10–12
	Advanced	3	12–15
Back Extensions on Exercise Ball	Beginner	1	8–10
	Intermediate	2	10–12
	Advanced	3	10–15

Stretch

EXERCISE	SETS	HOLD
One Leg Forward Flexion	3	15–60 Seconds
Hyper-Arch on Exercise Ball	3	15–60 Seconds
Spinal Twist	3	15–60 Seconds

CARDIOVASCUALR HEALTH: WEEK FIVE/ DAY 3

Aerobic

EXERCISE OPTIONS:	TIME:
Walking/Treadmill/Swimming/Biking/ Elliptical, Stairmaster/Aerobic	15 Minutes Heart Rate Goal: Between 70–85%

Strength Training: Lower and Upper Body

CHOOSE ONE EXERCISE FOR EACH BODY PART:

SETS AND REPS:

Beginner:
Sets: 1
Reps: 8–10

Intermediate:
Sets: 2
Reps: 10–12

Advanced:
Sets: 3
Reps: 12–15

Front of Legs
- Plié Squats Against Ball
- Seated Leg Extension
- Leg Extensions Using Ankle Weights
- Lying Bent Knee Leg Lifts*

Back of Legs
- Standing Hamstring Curls Using Ankle Weights
- Hamstring Curls Using Ankle Weights Over Bench, Chair or Ball
- Machine Hamstring Curls
- Standing Hamstring Curls*

Chest
- Ball Push-Ups
- Chest Press on Bench Using Body Bar or Smith Machine
- Dumbbell Presses Over Exercise Ball
- Wall Push-Ups*

Back
- Lat Pull-Downs
- One-Arm Kneeling Rows
- Machine Assisted Pull-Ups
- Back Rows*

*Equipment-Free Exercises

Core

EXERCISE	FITNESS LEVEL	SETS	REPS
Ball Crunches	Beginner	1	8–10
	Intermediate	2	10–12
	Advanced	3	10–15
Lateral Side Drops on Ball	Beginner	1	8–10
	Intermediate	2	10–12
	Advanced	3	12–15
Sitting Leg Lifts	Beginner	1	8–10
	Intermediate	2	10–12
	Advanced	3	10–15

Stretch

EXERCISE	SETS	HOLD
Hamstring Stretch: Single Leg Knee to Chest	3	15–60 Seconds
Piriformis Stretch	3	15–60 Seconds
Biceps/Triceps Stretches	3	15–60 Seconds

CARDIOVASCULAR HEALTH: WEEK FIVE/ DAY 4

Aerobic

EXERCISE OPTIONS:	TIME:
Walking/Treadmill/Swimming/Biking/ Elliptical, Stairmaster/Aerobic Video	40 Minutes Heart Rate Goal: Between 70–85%

Core

EXERCISE	FITNESS LEVEL	SETS	REPS
Isometric Squeezes	Beginner	1	8–10
	Intermediate	2	10–12
	Advanced	3	10–15
Pelvic Tilts	Beginner	1	8–10
	Intermediate	2	10–12
	Advanced	3	12–15
Crunches on Flat Bench Using Resistance Ball	Beginner	1	8–10
	Intermediate	2	10–12
	Advanced	3	10–15

Stretch

EXERCISE	SETS	HOLD
Spinal Twist	3	15–60 Seconds
Hyper-Arch on Exercise Ball	3	15–60 Seconds
Piriformis Stretch	3	15–60 Seconds

CARDIOVASCULAR HEALTH: WEEK FIVE/ DAY 5

Aerobic

EXERCISE OPTIONS:	TIME:
Walking/Treadmill/Swimming/Biking/ Elliptical, Stairmaster/Aerobic	15 Minutes Heart Rate Goal: Between 70–85%

Strength Training: Lower and Upper Body

CHOOSE ONE EXERCISE FOR EACH BODY PART:

SETS AND REPS:

Beginner:
Sets: 1
Reps: 8–10

Intermediate:
Sets: 2
Reps: 10–12

Advanced:
Sets: 3
Reps: 12–15

Glutes and Hips
- Ball Squats
- Side-Lying Leg Lifts Using Exercise Band
- Reverse Lunges Using Ankle Weights
- Sit Downs*

Calves
- Standing Heel Raises Using Dumbbells
- Machine Heel Raises
- Heel Raises*

Biceps
- Biceps Curls Using Dumbbells
- Body Bar Biceps Curls

- Cable Biceps Curls
- Isometric Biceps Curls*

Triceps
- Triceps Extensions Pull-Downs
- One-Arm Overhead Triceps Extension
- Lying Triceps Extension
- Triceps V-Backs*

Shoulders
- Side Arm Raises Using Dumbbells
- Overhead Presses Using Dumbbells
- Reverse Flyes on Ball Using Dumbbells
- Reverse Flyes*

*Equipment-Free Exercise

Core

EXERCISE	FITNESS LEVEL	SETS	REPS
Plank or Modified Plank	Beginner	1	8–10
	Intermediate	2	10–12
	Advanced	3	10–15
Ball Crunches	Beginner	1	8–10
	Intermediate	2	10–12
	Advanced	3	12–15
Kegels	Beginner	1	8–10
	Intermediate	2	10–12
	Advanced	3	10–15

Stretch

EXERCISE	SETS	HOLD
Hamstring Stretch: Single Leg Knee to Chest	3	15–60 Seconds
Quadriceps Stretch: Side-Lying Bent-Leg Stretch	3	15–60 Seconds
Hyper-Arch on Exercise Ball	3	15–60 Seconds

CARDIOVASCULAR HEALTH: WEEK FIVE/ DAY 6

Aerobic

EXERCISE OPTIONS:	TIME:
Walking/Treadmill/Swimming/Biking/ Elliptical, Stairmaster/Aerobic Video	40 Minutes Heart Rate Goal: Between 70–80%

Core

EXERCISE	FITNESS LEVEL	SETS	REPS
Leg Lifts	Beginner	1	8–10
	Intermediate	2	10–12
	Advanced	3	10–15
Kegels	Beginner	1	8–10
	Intermediate	2	10–12
	Advanced	3	12–15
Pelvic Tilts	Beginner	1	8–10
	Intermediate	2	10–12
	Advanced	3	10–15

Stretch

EXERCISE	SETS	HOLD
Hamstring Stretch: Single Leg Knee to Chest	3	15–60 Seconds
Hyper-Arch on Exercise Ball	3	15–60 Seconds
One Leg Forward Flexion	3	15–60 Seconds

CARDIOVASCULAR HEALTH: WEEK FIVE/ DAY 7
OPTIONAL: REST DAY

Aerobic

EXERCISE OPTIONS:	TIME:
Walking/Treadmill/Swimming/Biking/ Elliptical, Stairmaster/Aerobic Video	15 Minutes Heart Rate Goal: Between 65%–75%

Core

EXERCISE	FITNESS LEVEL	SETS	REPS
Classic Crunches	Beginner	1	8–10
	Intermediate	2	10–12
	Advanced	3	10–15
Cycle Rotations	Beginner	1	8–10
	Intermediate	2	10–12
	Advanced	3	12–15
Reverse Leg Lifts Using Ankle Weights	Beginner	1	8–10
	Intermediate	2	10–12
	Advanced	3	10–15

Stretch

EXERCISE	SETS	HOLD
Hamstring Stretch: Single Leg Knee to Chest	3	15–60 Seconds
Piriformis Stretch	3	15–60 Seconds
Spinal Twist	3	15–60 Seconds

CARDIOVASCULAR HEALTH : WEEK SIX/ DAY 1

Aerobic

EXERCISE OPTIONS:	TIME:
Walking/Treadmill/Swimming/Biking/ Elliptical, Stairmaster/Aerobic Video	40–45 Minutes Heart Rate Goal: Between 70%–85%

Core

EXERCISE	FITNESS LEVEL	SETS	REPS
Classic Crunches	Beginner	1	8–10
	Intermediate	2	10–12
	Advanced	3	10–15
Cycle Rotations	Beginner	1	8–10
	Intermediate	2	10–12
	Advanced	3	12–15
Reverse Leg Lifts Using Ankle Weights	Beginner	1	8–10
	Intermediate	2	10–12
	Advanced	3	10–15

Stretch

EXERCISE	SETS	HOLD
Hamstring Stretch: Single Leg Knee to Chest	3	15–60 Seconds
Piriformis Stretch	3	15–60 Seconds
Spinal Twist	3	15–60 Seconds

CARDIOVASCULAR HEALTH: WEEK SIX/ DAY 2

Aerobic

EXERCISE OPTIONS:	TIME:
Walking/Treadmill/Swimming/Biking/	40–45 Minutes
Elliptical, Stairmaster/Aerobic Video	Heart Rate Goal: Between 70–80%

Core

EXERCISE	FITNESS LEVEL	SETS	REPS
Reverse Leg Lifts with Ankle Weights	Beginner	1	8–10
	Intermediate	2	10–12
	Advanced	3	10–15
Cycle Rotations	Beginner	1	8–10
	Intermediate	2	10–12
	Advanced	3	12–15
Back Extensions on Exercise Ball	Beginner	1	8–10
	Intermediate	2	10–12
	Advanced	3	10–15

Stretch

EXERCISE	SETS	HOLD
One Leg Forward Flexion	3	15–60 Seconds
Hyper-Arch on Exercise Ball	3	15–60 Seconds
Spinal Twist	3	15–60 Seconds

CARDIOVASCULAR HEALTH: WEEK SIX/ DAY 3

Aerobic

EXERCISE OPTIONS:	TIME:
Walking/Treadmill/Swimming/Biking/ Elliptical, Stairmaster/Aerobic	15 Minutes Heart Rate Goal: Between 70–85%

Strength Training: Lower and Upper Body

CHOOSE ONE EXERCISE FOR EACH BODY PART:

SETS AND REPS:

Beginner:
Sets: 1
Reps: 8–10

Intermediate:
Sets: 2
Reps: 10–12

Advanced:
Sets: 3
Reps: 12–15

Front of Legs
- Plié Squats Against Ball
- Seated Leg Extension
- Leg Extensions Using Ankle Weights
- Lying Bent Knee Leg Lifts*

Back of Legs
- Standing Hamstring Curls Using Ankle Weights
- Hamstring Curls Using Ankle Weights Over Bench, Chair or Ball
- Machine Hamstring Curls
- Standing Hamstring Curls*

Chest
- Chest Flyes Using Dumbbells on Flat Bench
- Chest Press on Bench Using Body Bar or Smith Machine
- Dumbbell Presses Over Exercise Ball
- Floor Push-Ups*

Back
- Lat Pull-Downs
- One-Arm Kneeling Rows
- Bent-Over Body Bar Rows
- Arm Pull-Downs*

*Equipment-Free Exercise

Core

EXERCISE	FITNESS LEVEL	SETS	REPS
Plank or Modified Plank	Beginner	1	8–10
	Intermediate	2	10–12
	Advanced	3	10–15
Ball Crunches	Beginner	1	8–10
	Intermediate	2	10–12
	Advanced	3	12–15
Kegels	Beginner	1	8–10
	Intermediate	2	10–12
	Advanced	3	10–15

Stretch

EXERCISE	SETS	HOLD
Hamstring Stretch: Single Leg Knee to Chest	3	15–60 Seconds
Quadriceps Stretch: Side-Lying Bent-Leg Stretch	3	15–60 Seconds
Hyper-Arch on Exercise Ball	3	15–60 Seconds

CARDIOVASCULAR HEALTH: WEEK SIX/ DAY 4

Aerobic

EXERCISE OPTIONS:	TIME:
Walking/Treadmill/Swimming/Biking/ Elliptical, Stairmaster/Aerobic Video	40–45 Minutes Heart Rate Goal: Between 70%–85%

Core

EXERCISE	FITNESS LEVEL	SETS	REPS
Isometric Squeezes	Beginner	1	8–10
	Intermediate	2	10–12
	Advanced	3	10–15
Pelvic Tilts	Beginner	1	8–10
	Intermediate	2	10–12
	Advanced	3	12–15
Crunches on Flat Bench Using Resistance Ball	Beginner	1	8–10
	Intermediate	2	10–12
	Advanced	3	10–15

Stretch

EXERCISE	SETS	HOLD
Spinal Twist	3	15–60 Seconds
Hyper-Arch on Exercise Ball	3	15–60 Seconds
Piriformis Stretch	3	15–60 Seconds

CARDIOVASCULAR HEALTH: WEEK SIX/ DAY 5

Aerobic

EXERCISE OPTIONS:	TIME:
Walking/Treadmill/Swimming/Biking/ Elliptical, Stairmaster/Aerobic	15 Minutes Heart Rate Goal: Between 70–85%

Strength Training: Lower and Upper Body

CHOOSE ONE EXERCISE FOR EACH BODY PART:

SETS AND REPS:

Beginner:
Sets: 1
Reps: 8–10

Intermediate:
Sets: 2
Reps: 10–12

Advanced:
Sets: 3
Reps: 12–15

Glutes and Hips
- Ball Squats
- Side-Lying Leg Lifts Using Exercise Band
- Reverse Lunges Using Ankle Weights
- Sit Downs*

Calves
- Standing Heel Raises Using Dumbbells
- Machine Heel Raises
- Heel Raises*

Biceps
- Biceps Curls Using Dumbbells
- Seated One-Arm Biceps Curls

- Cable Biceps Curls
- Isometric Biceps Curls*

Triceps
- Triceps Extension Pull-Downs
- One-Arm Overhead Triceps Extension
- Lying Triceps Extension
- Triceps Wall Push-Ups*

Shoulders
- Angled One-Arm Side Raises
- Overhead Presses Using Dumbbells
- Reverse Flyes on Ball Using Dumbbells
- Reverse Flyes*

*Equipment-Free Exercise

Core

EXERCISE	FITNESS LEVEL	SETS	REPS
Back Extensions on Exercise Ball	Beginner	1	8–10
	Intermediate	2	10–12
	Advanced	3	10–15
Cycle Rotations	Beginner	1	8–10
	Intermediate	2	10–12
	Advanced	3	12–15
Sitting Leg Lifts	Beginner	1	8–10
	Intermediate	2	10–12
	Advanced	3	10–15

Stretch

EXERCISE	SETS	HOLD
One Leg Forward Flexion	3	15–60 Seconds
Piriformis Stretch	3	15–60 Seconds
Spinal Twist	3	15–60 Seconds

CARDIOVASCULAR HEALTH: WEEK SIX/ DAY 6

Aerobic

EXERCISE OPTIONS:	TIME:
Walking/Treadmill/Swimming/Biking/	40–45 Minutes
Elliptical, Stairmaster/Aerobic Video	Heart Rate Goal: Between 70%–85%

Core

EXERCISE	FITNESS LEVEL	SETS	REPS
Classic Crunches	Beginner	1	8–10
	Intermediate	2	10–12
	Advanced	3	10–15
Cycle Rotations	Beginner	1	8–10
	Intermediate	2	10–12
	Advanced	3	12–15
Reverse Leg Lifts Using Ankle Weights	Beginner	1	8–10
	Intermediate	2	10–12
	Advanced	3	10–15

Stretch

EXERCISE	SETS	HOLD
Hamstring Stretch: Single Leg Knee to Chest	3	15–60 Seconds
Piriformis Stretch	3	15–60 Seconds
Spinal Twist	3	15–60 Seconds

CARDIOVASCULAR HEALTH: WEEK SIX/ DAY 7
OPTIONAL: REST DAY

Aerobic

EXERCISE OPTIONS:	TIME:
Walking/Treadmill/Swimming/Biking/ Elliptical, Stairmaster/Aerobic Video	15 Minutes Heart Rate Goal: Between 70–85%

Core

EXERCISE	FITNESS LEVEL	SETS	REPS
Leg Lifts	Beginner	1	8–10
	Intermediate	2	10–12
	Advanced	3	10–15
Kegels	Beginner	1	8–10
	Intermediate	2	10–12
	Advanced	3	12–15
Pelvic Tilts	Beginner	1	8–10
	Intermediate	2	10–12
	Advanced	3	10–15

Stretch

EXERCISE	SETS	HOLD
Hamstring Stretch: Single Leg Knee to Chest	3	15–60 Seconds
Hyper-Arch on Exercise Ball	3	15–60 Seconds
One Leg Forward Flexion	3	15–60 Seconds

MASTER ANTI-AGING EXERCISE GRID

GOAL: Weight Loss, Tone, and Firm

	WEEK ONE	WEEK TWO	WEEK THREE	WEEK FOUR	WEEK FIVE	WEEK SIX
DAY 1	AEROBIC	AEROBIC	AEROBIC	AEROBIC	AEROBIC	AEROBIC
DAY 2	UPPER BODY	LOWER BODY	UPPER BODY	LOWER BODY	UPPER BODY	LOWER BODY
DAY 3	AEROBIC	AEROBIC	AEROBIC	AEROBIC	AEROBIC	AEROBIC
DAY 4	LOWER BODY	UPPER BODY	LOWER BODY	UPPER BODY	LOWER BODY	UPPER BODY
DAY 5	AEROBIC	AEROBIC	AEROBIC	AEROBIC	AEROBIC	AEROBIC
DAY 6	UPPER BODY	LOWER BODY	UPPER BODY	LOWR BODY	UPPER BODY	LOWER BODY
DAY 7	AEROBIC	AEROBIC	AEROBIC	AEROBIC	AEROBIC	AEROBIC

GOAL: Increase Strength, Tone, and Firm

	WEEK ONE	WEEK TWO	WEEK THREE	WEEK FOUR	WEEK FIVE	WEEK SIX
DAY 1	UPPER BODY	UPPER BODY	UPPER BODY	UPPER BODY	UPPER BODY	UPPER BODY
DAY 2	AEROBIC	AEROBIC	AEROBIC	AEROBIC	AEROBIC	AEROBIC
DAY 3	LOWER BODY	LOWER BODY	LOWER BODY	LOWER BODY	LOWER BODY	LOWER BODY
DAY 4	AEROBIC	AEROBIC	AEROBIC	AEROBIC	AEROBIC	AEROBIC
DAY 5	UPPER BODY	UPPER BODY	UPPER BODY	UPPER BODY	UPPER BODY	UPPER BODY
DAY 6	AEROBIC	AEROBIC	AEROBIC	AEROBIC	AEROBIC	AEROBIC
DAY 7	LOWER BODY	LOWER BODY	LOWER BODY	LOWER BODY	LOWER BODY	LOWER BODY

GOAL: Cardiovascular Health, Tone, and Firm

	WEEK ONE	WEEK TWO	WEEK THREE	WEEK FOUR	WEEK FIVE	WEEK SIX
DAY 1	AEROBIC	AEROBIC	AEROBIC	AEROBIC	AEROBIC	AEROBIC
DAY 2	AEROBIC	AEROBIC	AEROBIC	AEROBIC	AEROBIC	AEROBIC
DAY 3	LOWER & UPPER	LOWER & UPPER	LOWER & UPPER	LOWER & UPPER	LOWER & UPPER	LOWER & UPPER
DAY 4	AEROBIC	AEROBIC	AEROBIC	AEROBIC	AEROBIC	AEROBIC
DAY 5	LOWER & UPPER	LOWER & UPPER	LOWER & UPPER	LOWER & UPPER	LOWER & UPPER	LOWER & UPPER
DAY 6	AEROBIC	AEROBIC	AEROBIC	AEROBIC	AEROBIC	AEROBIC
DAY 7	AEROBIC	AEROBIC	AEROBIC	AEROBIC	AEROBIC	AEROBIC

APPENDICES

MY HEALTH-LIFE MISSION STATEMENT

I _____ am _____ years of age. Today's date is: _____

I feel my health and body are _____ because _____

I know if I follow both the Anti-Aging Exercise Strategies and Life Balancing Exercises in *Muscle Your Way Through Menopause*, I will

_____

_____

My top 3 Body Preserving goals are:

1. _____
2. _____
3. _____

My top 3 Life Balancing goals are:

1. _____
2. _____
3. _____

It has been _____ for me to achieve these goals in the past because _____

I am starting this health- and life-altering journey today because I want to _____

_____

_____

My Health-Life Mission and my Personal Promise to myself is: _____

_____

_____

HOW MANY CALORIES DO I BURN?

The chart below gives you the approximate amount of kcals you burn in 30 minutes performing various exercises and activities. For example, if you weigh 120 pounds and you're doing medium intensity aerobics, you will burn about 169 kcals for your 30 minutes of exercise.

Weight in Pounds

	100	105	110	115	120	125	130	135	140	145	150	155	160	165
Doing Dumbbells	117	123	129	134	141	147	152	158	164	170	176	182	188	194
Aerobics Medium	140	147	154	162	169	176	183	190	197	204	211	218	225	232
Aerobics High Intensity	184	193	202	212	221	230	239	249	258	267	276	285	295	304
Cycling Outdoors	136	143	150	157	164	170	177	184	191	198	205	211	218	225
Stationary Bike	87	91	96	100	105	109	113	117	122	127	131	135	140	144
Jogging	184	193	203	212	221	230	239	249	258	267	276	285	295	304
Jumping Rope	220	231	243	254	266	276	287	298	309	320	331	342	353	365
Swimming	212	223	234	244	255	266	277	287	298	308	319	330	340	351
Tennis	148	156	163	171	178	186	193	201	208	216	223	230	238	245
Walking	117	123	129	135	141	147	152	158	164	170	177	182	188	195
Water Aerobics	90	94.5	99	104	108	113	117	122	126	131	135	140	144	149
Yoga/Pilates	90	94.5	99	104	108	113	117	122	126	131	135	140	144	149

	170	175	180	185	190	195	200	205	210	215	220	225	230	235
Doing Dumbbells	199	205	211	217	223	229	235	240	246	252	258	264	270	276
Aerobics Medium	239	246	253	260	267	274	281	288	295	302	309	316	323	330
Aerobics Intense	313	322	331	341	350	359	368	377	387	396	405	414	423	433
Cycling Outdoors	232	239	245	252	259	266	273	280	286	293	300	307	314	320
Stationary Bike	148	153	157	161	166	170	175	179	183	188	192	196	201	205
Jogging	313	322	331	341	350	359	368	377	387	396	405	414	423	433
Jumping Rope	376	387	398	409	420	431	442	453	464	475	486	497	509	519
Swimming	362	372	383	394	404	415	425	436	447	457	468	479	489	450
Tennis	253	260	268	275	282	290	297	305	312	320	327	334	342	350
Walking	199	205	211	217	223	229	235	240	246	252	258	264	270	276
Water Aerobics	153	158	162	167	171	176	180	185	189	194	198	203	207	212
Yoga/Pilates	153	158	162	167	171	176	180	185	189	194	198	203	207	212

ACKNOWLEDGMENTS

The question writers are asked more frequently than any other is: "Where did you get the idea for that...book, story, screenplay, poem?" The truth is ideas are easy to come by. The trick, of course, is making those ideas come to life and, if that weren't difficult enough, finding advocates, other than your loved ones, who think you are onto something special and the only one who possesses the talent to execute it.

In the case of *Muscle Your Way Through Menopause...and Beyond*, its first real friend came in the form of my stalwart agent Kirsten Manges. Beautiful inside and out, from our first meeting she believed in me and my message, and worked tirelessly to make this book a reality. Some working relationships feel organic from the start...and if you're blessed, they turn into wonderful friendships as well.

This leads me to my book's second great friend, my editor Marnie Cochran. She accepted, supported, advised, edited with prudence and keen intelligence, has been a bountiful cheerleader, and most importantly, gave me creative freedom and her inherent trust.

A special thank you goes to Dr. Philip Brooks, who not only wrote the foreword, but gave me invaluable assistance during another profound event in my life, the birth of my first child, my daughter, three decades ago. For both my cherished daughter, and the words in the foreword, I am forever and truly grateful.

In remembrance of my parents, my mother, Selma Ludwin Sherman, who instilled in me a belief in myself telling me always, "There is nothing you can't do if you set your heart to it." Beautiful and smart, adored wife of my father Marvin, a whiz at grammar and one of the best spellers I ever knew—she taught me the value and power of the written word and if that weren't good enough, how to traverse the aging process with incomparable grace and beauty. And my father, Marvin, who is genetically responsible for two of my most valued assets: my physical strength and my sense of humor.

Also in memory of my dear friend Wendy Woskoff, a woman of indomitable spirit and bountiful heart, who left us much, much too soon. She is missed, and thought of, everyday.

Hugs and kisses and endless gratitude to my to my dear ones: Nancy Marks, Lori Milken, Jill Chozen, Hillari Koppelman, Carole Robbins, Carla Kirkeby, Katherine Hughes Del Tufo and Ellen Sandler, because we've shared most of everything in our lives that has ever had any meaning and if we didn't, it didn't mean very much anyway.

A woman does not live by female friends alone, so thank you to my chevaliers and knights: Philip Gary Miller, who listens to me when I need to be listened to; Howard Marks who always advises me when I need advice; Russell Stein, who cheers me up and knows when I need cheering; Mitchell Ohlbaum and Norman Steinberg, who make me laugh and equally important, laugh at me when I need to be laughed at.

And, once again, nothing I have ever accomplished or hope to accomplish would have the least bit of meaning if not for my treasured and adored children, of whom their father would be unspeakably proud: Samantha, a beautiful and amazing young woman whose successes are only exceeded by her sweetness of heart and goodness of nature; and Bennett, who, at twenty-one, probably wishes his name was not being mentioned in a book for women about menopause, but who is beyond exceptional in every way and I'm sure will forgive me.

INDEX OF EXERCISES